THE HILL OF SEVEN COLORS

DOMINIQUE HOFFMAN

Zizania Productions

THE HILL OF SEVEN COLORS

This is a work of fiction. Names, characters, places and events are wholly the products of the author's imagination, and any resemblance to actual business establishments, events or locations is entirely coincidental.

ISBN: 979-8-9905024-1-3 (Paperback)
ISBN: 979-8-9905024-0-6 (Ebook)

Cover art by Wilbert Sweet (**www.artstation.com/will**)

Zizania Productions
dominique@zizania.com

THE HILL OF SEVEN COLORS

1 - Learning to Dive Without Fins

Splattered white lumps cover the roof of my car. I glare up at a line of birds perched on an electrical wire. "I feed you every day and this is how you thank me."

I go back inside and return with a bottle of water and a sponge. Watching me scrub, my neighbor, Ron, laughs.

"It's because you washed the car. They always poop on shiny cars."

Ron is a Vietnam veteran. He regularly walks up and down the street, never without a can of beer in hand, even at this hour of the morning. He keeps watch on everyone and everything, mi-voyeur, mi-protector.

I rinse off the smeared paste and drive to work.

As I open my office door, the phone rings, an international number. I ignore it—probably spam. It rings again with the same number. Maybe it's a patient overseas who needs help. Rare, but it happens.

"Hindsight Therapy. How may I help you?"

"May I speak to Dr. Saylor, please?" A light Spanish accent.

"Speaking."

"This is Daniel from the scuba diving group. Do you remember?"

A pang punches my insides; I breathe deep before answering. "Yes... yes, of course. Huh, how are you?" It's unexpected, unreal. The man I was so infatuated with for a week on a vacation resort a month ago, a man who never even asked for my email address. I take another deep breath.

"I'm fine. How've you been?" he says with poise.

"Goo-good. How did you get my number?"

"You told me you were a therapist, so, I googled you. Google said there is only one beautiful therapist and scuba diver in the United States."

I tremble and scratch my neck. "Haha. You want money or information?"

"Information. I want to know if you find me irresistible, like most women."

"Is that what your mother told you?"

"That hurts. Let me wipe off the blood. I was calling because..." He pauses for what seems like an hour.

"...I miss you. We had such a good time in Mexico. When is your next scuba trip?"

My heart flips. My neck itches as it always does when I'm nervous. I fold my hand into a fist to avoid scratching and rub the skin with my knuckles.

"It depends on how this virus situation develops. Lot of countries have closed their borders already. Just a matter of time before we follow suit."

"There is a solution now. Just get an injection of Ayudín."

"What's Ayudín?"

"I think it's called Clorox over there. Your president's recommendation."

I blush on behalf of the United States of America. "I'm sorry the world had to hear that."

"Hey, serves you right. You inflicted Madonna on us. As if the people of Argentina haven't suffered enough."

Caught off guard, I almost stutter in my response. "I think the US already apologized for that." We laugh in unison.

Before we hang up, he asks to meet over Zoom that evening. For a woman, video is a tremendous disadvantage. We can't showcase our beautiful clothes or shoes. It's all about words and facial expressions. Nevertheless, I agree to meet him digitally.

My head is dizzy, and my body feels heavy, similar to a change in barometric pressure at the advent of a storm.

Having shared my infatuation with my friend, Tina, I text her to share the news.

Tina, guess what?

??

The guy I met on the scuba diving trip just called.

Really? Better find out what he's hiding. Maybe he's a mafioso.

He's from Argentina not Italy.

Soccer fanatic. Just as bad.

You're jealous. I'm about to date someone dark and handsome, and you're stuck with a gringo.

Let's see if I can sing it. 'Watch out for Annie, Argentina.'

Joking aside, he's so imposing, makes me feel like a child.

You, intimidated? I'd pay to see that. I wanna b u! You have a FUNtastic career, ur athletic, and have an exotic lover.

He's not my lover yet.

I wrap up my work early and hurry home. I lost interest in going to the kickboxing class I planned to attend. I probably won't enjoy it. I've been getting strange bouts of pain in the arm for a week, which are now escalating to headaches.

/\ /\ /\

I open the computer half an hour before our scheduled date. As I wait in front of the screen, I can't describe what I feel as butterflies—more like birds flying everywhere under my skin. A PhD. in psychology is useless in a dating setting with such a charismatic man. I check my face in the mirror once more, then sit back in front of the camera, stretch my neck and shoulders, and breathe deep. I want him to see a confident and poised woman, but my neck is heating again. Part of me wants to turn off the computer. What kind of relationship can I have with someone in a different time zone? But images of us together in Mexico, his protective gestures underwater, and his smile haunt me. The mind submits to the heart.

His name comes on the screen, followed by his smile. My knees shake; I scratch my neck and quickly put my hand on the desk. He's different from the way I remember. A suit and tie, hair neatly combed back, revealing a receding hairline and a broad forehead. He's sitting comfortably, leaned back against a tall chair. I like his round shoulders. Unlike square arrogant ones, bony and penurious ones, or tired saggy ones, round shoulders are elegant yet inviting and snuggly. His hands are folded on the desk. It's a large desk with a shiny surface, a pencil cup and a vase without flowers in the corner.

I check my face on the screen, put a hand on my neck, and tilt my head to the left to avoid the camera distortion.

"So good to see you again." He pauses before continuing. "I feel like it's been years."

"Are you saying you forgot what I look like?"

"That's impossible."

"Can you believe how much this pandemic has changed our lives in just a month? It's like the entire world is in mourning."

"Most devastating for the tourism industry and airlines. All my trips have been canceled."

"How often do you travel?"

"I go to the UK about every six weeks."

"So, what do you do in Buenos Aires, aside from tango dancing?"

"Tango shows are everywhere. There are also plays, open-air concerts. Buenos Aires is a European city. A lot of the architecture is similar to Paris or Madrid. Amazing museums, too."

My chest tightens. Images of crowds dancing, shopping, and sipping beverages at café terraces stream before my eyes. He's so far away, in a fun lively town, while I live in dormitory Reston. I clear my throat. "Best museums are in Washington, DC."

"Why is that?"

"They're free."

"I remember. A great place for a student to take a date."

I put on my best smile and throw that fishing rod again. "So, how many girlfriends do you have in Buenos Aires?"

If you're married, this is a good time to tell me.

"Hard to count. Women can't keep their hands off of me. That's why I rarely socialize."

"I didn't mean imaginary."

He shakes his head and laughs. With the agility of a fencer, he turns the conversation back to me. "Tell me about the type of patients you counsel."

"I counsel couples and patients with trauma. I'm actually

writing a book about the effects of PTSD on families. The majority of treatments focus on the patient, though family members are also affected, but they're hardly ever included. Basically, I'd like a holistic approach to the treatment of trauma victims."

"Amazing. When do you plan to publish?"

"It'll take a while. I'm in the research phase."

"Have you published before?"

"Two books. One about children of narcissists and another about spouses of PTSD patients. Most of my work is about trauma in all its forms."

While we're discussing my professional endeavors, my mind is racing to find questions that will unveil his secret, the one I suspected he was hiding from the first time we met.

"Do you like opera?" he asks.

"Not really. Women always die at the end. Even when they're brave and smart like Norma or Tosca, they never triumph. Why d'you ask?"

"I have a relative who's a famous opera singer. She moved to Europe in the eighties."

"Type her name in the chat. I'll check her out."

Once again, I give more than I receive. Maybe he's in the middle of a divorce or a separation. It can't be marriage. He's talking to me late at night from his home. I'll find out soon enough.

Λ Λ Λ

For the next three weeks following our first digital date, I wake up every morning eager to check WhatsApp. There's always a message waiting for me. We develop a ritual of video dates on Tuesday evenings, phone calls Saturday mornings, and daily texts. Paradoxically, it's old-fashioned dating: communication before consummation.

On this Tuesday, we start our conversation as usual by relating the events of our day. Then we move to other topics, some flirting, some vague plans to meet in the future. He interrupts me just before I tell him about my new difficult patient.

He looks over his left shoulder. “I need to end our session early today.” He hesitates, then looks at the camera. “I have to pick up Tanya.” The words fly out of his mouth in one burst.

“Your girlfriend?”

“My daughter,” he says with a wry smile.

“Oh, how old?”

“She’s fifteen and loves theater. She’s in a school play.”

A chill rushes down my spine. I ask for pictures, which he happily displays on the screen. Tanya is a slender teenager with long brown hair swinging below her shoulders. She has a slightly oval face with dark blue eyes. I distinctly see her father in her. They share the same winsome smile.

As he moves through the photo album, I notice Tanya is often standing next to a woman in a sophisticated tilt-in-space wheelchair. Having worked in hospitals with car accident victims, I know it’s a wheelchair used mainly by quadriplegics.

“She’s beautiful. Who’s the lady in the wheelchair?”

“That’s my wife.”

Silence. The type of silence that follows an earthquake. The ceiling has fallen on my head and the dust from the blast rushes in to coat my mouth. I catch my breath but don’t have any words. I want to hide or run away. I’ll figure out how I feel later.

“I need to get going, too. I promised my dad I’d call him. It was his birthday yesterday.” Instead of turning off the video, I stand to prepare my exit.

“Annie. Sit down, please.”

I freeze. He’s able to chain me to the chair with the power of his voice through a computer screen. The way he says my name sounds like a command. I sit but can’t look him in the eyes. After a few seconds of suffocating silence, I finally grab the few crumbs of courage I have left and mumble, “I can’t get involved with a married man.”

“I know that. You’re not involved with anything.”

Heat scorches in a wave over my face and my neck itches again. I scratch; the rash turns into buds. “What’s going on between us, exactly?”

He lowers his eyes and frowns. It only makes him sexier. He’s struggling to find an appropriate reply, so I throw him a lifebuoy and ask in a softer voice, “I thought you were single. So, what’s the story?”

“If you’re looking for a simple answer, life doesn’t always offer those. I’m not some married man looking for action.”

He has probably rehearsed this scene many times in his head.

“When Tanya was about five, Nina fell from a horse and was left paralyzed from the neck down.”

“How devastating.”

“It was, but we changed our life to adapt. Nina wanted everything to be normal for Tanya...”

“Huh...” It’s obvious he wants to say more. Instead, he rubs his chin and looks sideways. Emotion rises in his words as he relives the accident and the months that followed.

“Did you reach out to anyone else?”

“Never. I was completely devoted to her. I hired a governess to take care of the household and drive Tanya to ballet lessons or whatever she needed, and we maintained a normal family life.”

With a twinge in my gut, I ask, “Are you still close?”

“A couple of years ago, her health declined, and she was put on dialysis. She became more and more distant from everyone and a bit hostile toward me. She rarely said anything and smiled only when Tanya was around.”

“Did you try to get her into therapy?”

“One evening, we were watching a movie, and this actress was running in a swimsuit. I made a lame comment like, ‘With legs like that, she can swim across the ocean.’ She snapped, which was out of character, and yelled, ‘You want a girl with legs? Then you’d better look somewhere else!’

Next day, she asked for a divorce; she said she no longer loved me and accused me of staying with her out of duty. Doctors said it was probably depression and to give it time. Months went by; her resolve remained the same. Any time I went to see her, she'd turn her head away and close her eyes. We agreed that a divorce would not be good for Tanya, so I offered a separation where we lived in the same house, on separate floors."

"I'm sorry. That's gotta be lonely. How did Tanya take it?"

"It was rough at the beginning, but we learned to adapt."

I struggled to formulate the next question. "How's... your wife now?"

"Still withdrawn. And her health continues to decline."

Is distance my most attractive feature? No need to sneak around when dating someone in another country. All kinds of thoughts shoot through my mind like arrows: end the Zoom session now; finish the session and never talk to him again; tell him I'm angry. I disable the camera and mute myself to exhale, stretch my arms, and lower my head between my elbows.

"Annie? Are you still there?"

I regain my composure and face the camera again. "I'm sure you met a lot of women over the years. Why me?"

"I think what you're asking is if this is the first time I reach out to a woman."

"There are plenty of beautiful women in Buenos Aires."

"There are. When you're dealing with this kind of situation, every day revolves around that person. The last thing on your mind is fooling around. But now we have minimal contact. She no longer cares what I do, but still, I wasn't actively looking." He lowers his gaze and smiles with hesitation. "Hmm... From the first time I talked to you, I knew I could fall in love with you. Your wit, your sense of humor, and your beauty are an unusual combination to find in one woman."

"Not to mention my legs."

"See what I mean? I tried to forget you when I came back from Mexico, but the joy I felt when being around you wouldn't fade. I wrestled with the decision to contact you; partly because I have so little to offer. But also, I exchanged vows with someone else. I talked it over with a couple of friends and my priest. Everyone agreed that under these circumstances, I should pursue happiness. I'd like to have you in my life, but a divorce is not an option for me."

"I understand."

"Annie... I would not be contacting someone thousands of miles away if I didn't believe you were special. But I also made a promise I intend to keep."

Once we say our goodbyes, I close the laptop and stare at the window. I turn on the lights and slowly parse the new data. I'm not ready to let go, but I don't know how to hold on.

Λ Λ Λ

A month earlier...

With my PADI in hand, I was ready to explore the waters of Riviera Maya. February was the perfect time to escape to Mexico. Most diving resorts are in the middle of nowhere, but Riviera Maya was a hidden treasure. Our small resort was surrounded by water and covered with luscious greenery under a blue and cloud-free sky.

I was scared on the first diving day. Leaving my comfortable world for an unknown, dangerous one terrified me. But the promise of beauty and discovery still drew me in. Once I reached the water, I filled my lungs with air and pushed downward. At first, I couldn't see anything in the murky depths, but the sun's rays penetrated enough to illuminate the hidden world.

Everything we take for granted on land—breathing, moving, the noises we ignore—are all amplified underwater, and nothing is left to chance. Every movement takes effort and precision. One moment of inattention could mean death. Nature has strict rules and doesn't forgive.

We followed the diving master through cliffs of coral, small and large plants, and so many colorful fish with fluorescent blue, bright yellow, and light orange. Entire schools zigzagged around us; a few chased each other; occasionally, a thin gray creature burrowed in the ocean floor and disappeared.

Sometimes, I dragged my fins, earning a reprimand from the diving master. In the vast and mighty space lived a fragile ecosystem. We were instructed to stay clear of plants and not to disturb the ocean floor, so little critters could thrive in their own home.

On the second diving day, after we returned to the boat, everyone moved to the uncovered benches to perfect their tans and check their cell phones. I headed to the tray of oranges. I filled a small plate and sat in the shade, glancing upward when suddenly approached by a handsome man dripping with saltwater. He asked why I was sitting alone.

"Sun doesn't like me much," I said after swallowing a mouthful of orange.

"You burn? Are you Irish?"

I looked at him with a question mark on my face.

"Very white skin and red hair," he said.

"The skin was free. The hair was on sale."

He laughed and extended his hand for me to shake. "I'm Daniel."

"Annie."

His eyes scanned me from head to toe, so I returned the favor. I started with his hands, pleased by the absence of jewelry. A couple of hairs on his beautifully sculpted chest competed for territory, above a timid protrusion of his belly.

"How long have you been diving?" I asked.

"Ten years. You?"

"This is my first dive. I just got certified."

"I noticed. You were floating."

"I think I'm too tall to be buoyant. I saw a fish laugh."

"You just need more practice."

When we returned to land, we walked in separate directions toward our bungalows.

The next day, I was the first to arrive at the diving shop. Other divers came shortly after, but no Daniel. While my diving mates dressed in their suits, applied sunscreen and chatted away, my eyes were fixated on the entrance. Had I hallucinated a handsome diver? I put on my suit and followed the crowd to the boat and dove with a little more confidence but with a dint in my joy.

On the third day, I joined the divers at the diving shop again—not without hope of running into him. A spark of lightning traveled through my body when I spotted him chatting with another diver. As I approached, he turned and gave me a cheerful smile, interrupting his conversation to greet me.

"Annie! How are you this morning?"

I lifted my chin. "My diving skills improved during your day off." I immediately regretted my response.

He moved toward me. "Not as much as they'll improve today under my leadership."

We walked together to the boat; he helped me put on my gear, and we sat next to each other while waiting for the signal to dive. The boat rocked gently on the calm dark-blue ocean, taking in the soft sunlight of the morning.

"Cross your ankles to keep your legs together when you enter the water," he said.

"Nobody told me that in the training."

"Got any spit?"

I frowned in response.

"It's a product you apply on your mask to prevent fogging." He pulled out a little bottle from his bag and squeezed a drop of the sticky substance into my mask. He smeared it with his finger and dipped the mask in the bucket of water.

"On the captain's count, you want to jump without hesitation. Otherwise, you can get hurt."

He put his hand on my shoulder, and my fear evaporated. I wanted to make him proud, so I tucked my chin in my chest, crossed my ankles, and when the captain said, "Three," I fell backward.

Underwater, he kept me close. He helped me with my buoyancy and reminded me not to use my arms. At some point, he stood in front of me and crossed my arms over my chest so I'd stop swimming. He gestured to a fish, then at my fins as to say, *"Fish don't have arms. Use your fins."* I turned into an obedient student. What woman wouldn't want the protection and guidance of a handsome Poseidon?

After the dive, we took off our suits, and I sat in the shade, watching him shower. The water dripped smoothly on his bronze skin. My eyes locked on his arms and I wondered what it would be like to have them hold me. I shook my head to repudiate the thought. I barely knew the man. *Slow down, Annie.*

I pulled a towel from my bag to put over my hair, which now looks nappy; combing it wouldn't help. I smeared a dollop of sunscreen on my face to keep the freckles from invading.

"Freckles? Beautiful," he said as he sat next to me.

"Don't say that. It encourages them."

"They only come out in the sun?"

"They think it's an invitation to party."

/\ /\ /\

Every evening, he knocked at my door to accompany me to dinner with the group. We sat together at the restaurant, surrounded by other divers, but our conversation had the intimacy of schoolmates.

When the waitress came, he addressed her in Spanish and often ordered a burrito stuffed with rice, beans, avocado, salsa, a tray of sautéed vegetables, or some other meatless dish. One evening, I inquired about his food choice.

"Are you vegetarian?"

He put his arm on the back of my chair and talked to me in a lower voice, our heads almost touching. "Nooo," he said with a sarcastic glare and half a smile.

From the look on his face, I'd violated some sacred diet-labeling law.

"Vegan. The term vegetarian is corrupt."

"I will never vote for it."

"Cute," he said with the most radiant smile I'd ever seen.

I leaned back against the chair, my back touching his hand. I threw a bundle of hair behind my shoulder and caught his gaze on my neck. "Why don't vegetarians go to the gym with vegans?"

"There is no cheese at the gym?"

"The relationship won't work out."

"You're funny." He swallowed a gulp of his margarita. "And what do you call a person who doesn't eat meat but eats cheese?"

"A vegetarian?" I answered.

"A hypocrite."

"I didn't know vegans had a sense of humor."

"That's the reputation. You know, vegetarians are a pain. They make it difficult for us in restaurants because everyone assumes we eat cheese and eggs. It's worse overseas. In France, restaurants won't even talk to someone who doesn't indulge in French cuisine where everything is smothered in crême fraiche. Spanish vegan restaurants serve fish. In Korea, the word vegan hasn't made it into the vocabulary yet."

"I'm sorry your dietary struggles span several countries. Are you a vegan spy using architect as a cover?"

"I work for a British company." He winked.

To keep the peace, I ordered meatless dishes, too.

"So, how's that wall going?" he asked.

I rolled my eyes and cocked my head in his direction. "Slow. Construction workers are unreliable."

"Sorry, I couldn't resist."

I pressed on my chili relleno with a fork; warm, gooey

cheese oozed on the plate. "Is your family from Buenos Aires?" I asked, probing into his marital status.

"My grandfather is from Spain, actually. My grandmother is Polish. She came to Argentina during the Second World War."

I twisted a lock of hair behind my ear. "Your grandmother was Jewish?"

"Polish. Just as bad as far as the Nazis were concerned. A lot of Europeans, mainly Jews, came to Argentina just before the war. It was particularly rough for Jewish women..."

He drifted into the history of Argentina during World War II, and I was left without the answer I wanted. The absence of a ring did not always equate singlehood.

I lifted my chin and shot my next question like a fisherman throwing a line into a lake. "Aside from working, what do you do for entertainment?"

"There is plenty of activity in Buenos Aires, but I don't go out much. I travel quite a bit. So, when I'm home, I like to relax. When the weather is nice, I play tennis. Do you know what we don't have in Argentina?"

"Donald Trump?"

He sighed. "We have much worse, I'm afraid."

"So, what's missing in Argentina?"

"Amusement parks—with roller coasters."

"Is that what you like to do for fun?"

"Not exactly, but that's why a lot of Argentines go to Florida."

He smiled then. Some kind of key opened my heart, so many warm sensations rushed in. Something about the way he laughed with a velvety voice, the way he curled his lips. To avoid staring, I turned my head to the door. A svelte woman with a proud bust entered. I caught him looking.

"Enjoying the view?" I asked.

"Not really. Lacks freckles."

"Flattery will get you nowhere, my friend."

After dinner, he walked me to my bungalow along the marina, guided by the glowing lights of the boats and a star-dotted sky. We walked side by side and stopped to look at the rippling multicolor light effects on the water. He moved his hand toward mine but retrieved it immediately.

"That would make a great painting," he said.

"You paint?"

"Used to." He put his hand on my shoulder to guide me away from the marina and resume walking. Lightning sparks traveled down my spine.

"Why did you stop painting?"

He ran his hand on my forearm. "Long story. We'll save it for another scuba trip."

He wished me good night at my doorstep and walked away. Once inside, I rushed to my laptop and combed the internet for his profile. LinkedIn was his only online presence. He'd been an architect for years and worked on many international projects for which he won several awards.

/\ /\ /\

For our last evening in Mexico, Daniel invited me to dinner without the group. I was certain we would exchange contact information—maybe even a kiss.

It was still daylight when he knocked at my door. I quivered when I saw him through the window. He was elegantly dressed in black pants and a light gray shirt. His shiny hair combed back with ringlets covering his neck. I wore a light pink blouse and a long white silk skirt with flats. I didn't want to be taller than him. He was six feet tall but, with my five feet nine and high heels, I was always taller than most men.

"You look stunning," he said when I opened the door. He leaned over to kiss me on the cheek. He had a light about him that drew me in further every time we interacted.

We walked side by side to the restaurant. Every woman who crossed our path scrutinized him. One of them was looking so intently that she tripped. She noticed me and we exchanged a smile. Unaware of the attention he was generating, he focused on the marina, trying to identify the most interesting yachts.

We arrived at a restaurant by the marina and the hostess sat us at a cozy table overlooking the boats. Daniel pulled out a chair for me and sat down after I did, then opened the wine list.

"Are you familiar with Argentinian wines?"

"I know two wines: Chardonnay and Chianti."

"Tonight, you'll learn a third one. I can't let you leave without introducing you to Argentinian wines. What's your favorite dessert?"

"Key lime pie."

He waved the waitress to our table and a long conversation in Spanish ensued.

"Did you negotiate a new trade treaty?" I asked after the waitress left.

"I ordered a Malbec from Mendoza called Catena Alta. It's not on the menu because they have only one bottle left."

"And you ordered it for us?"

"Yes," he said with the certainty of a man who's used to being in charge. "It has a fruity flavor, a hint of acidity, but slides on the palate like velvet. I think you'll like it. And because it's light, it complements well-seasoned vegan dishes."

The evening had fallen. The lights of the marina, and the dim glow of the restaurant created the perfect romantic, dreamy atmosphere. While he tried to initiate me to Argentinian wines, and as my eyes stared at him, his voice undulated in my head like a melody. I floated a little above the ground. His face was smooth, without wrinkles, except for a few lines on his forehead, giving him an intellectual stamp. I always found wrinkles sexy on a man. Thick eyebrows accentuated wide green eyes filled with curiosity and playful sparks when he looked at me.

"So, how did you end up in Virginia from Oregon?"

"I went to Harvard. After graduation, I wanted to move to a warmer state. On January 2, I drove down to Virginia. It was snowing in New England. Once I passed Delaware and got closer to Maryland, the sun was shining so bright, I put on sunglasses and took off my parka. The next day, I went to work in short sleeves."

"What made you go into psychology?"

"I was always fascinated by the functions of the brain. I first wanted to study neurology. But I didn't want to spend years in residency."

"No childhood trauma?"

"I see." I waved a hand in dismissal. "You thought I went into psychology because I was crazy?"

"Not at all." He frowned and shook his head. "Lots of people go into a profession because of previous experience. I apologize, I meant no offense."

I tilted my head and smiled. "None taken. I was just pulling your chain. But you're correct, it's the general assumption. I take it you don't believe in psychotherapy."

He winked. "I believe in *you*."

I moved my face closer to his and leered. "Nice try. So, what's the secret?"

"What secret?"

I grinned. "You're hiding something."

The waitress brought the bottle of wine, opened it, and poured him a sample. After he approved it, she filled our glasses and went to the next table. He lifted his glass and looked me in the eyes. "To the most beautiful evening of the year."

"The year has just begun." As soon as I said it, I realized I had killed the moment.

His eyes wandered to the rippling streaks of light on the water, then back at me pensively. "It won't get better than this." We filled our mouths with wine.

"What made you study building drawing?"

He smiled and nodded his head, looking me straight in the eyes. "Touché."

Uncomfortable with his gaze, I occupied my hands by pulling my hair back and rolling it into a bun.

"I like you better with your hair down. Is it naturally curly?"

"Yes, it's a curse." I sip on the wine before moving to more personal questions. "So, where about in Buenos Aires do you live?"

"Ricoletta. Are you familiar with Buenos Aires?" He opened his phone and scrolled through pictures, mainly of buildings, parks with giant trees resembling sequoias, monuments, but no family pictures.

"Actually, I grew up in La Plata, near Buenos Aires. As a matter of fact, La Plata is the capital city of the Buenos Aires Province."

"So, do you have any siblings?" he asked.

"I'm an only child. I'm actually adopted."

He raises his eyebrows. "Fascinating. I hear parents who adopt bond with the child the same way they do their own."

"My parents certainly do. How about you? "

"I have a sister. She also lives in Buenos Aires and has two children."

It was a perfect segue to ask if he had children, but a loud couple approached and asked us to take pictures of them with their dessert. The woman had a smile that competed with Julia Roberts'. "It's our honeymoon." She beamed. Then they wanted to take a picture of us with them. Daniel politely declined the offer.

After dinner, he walked me to my bungalow, but he was quieter than usual. Our synchronized steps echoed on the cobblestones. As we turned into the path leading to my "habitacion", he finally broke the oppressive silence.

"What's your last name?"

"Saylor."

His hand brushed my arm. "Annie Saylor from Virginia. What time is your flight tomorrow?"

"Eleven in the morning. Daniel Lorenzo from Argentina." We shared our last chuckle and he put his hand on my shoulder. It was enough to lift me into the clouds like a lost feather flying aimlessly in the breeze.

Then there was the most blatant sign of indifference: no mention of staying in touch. I landed from my cloud like a plane in a storm. My feminine intuition and my clinical education told me he was interested. But his behavior was of a man with a secret, and I was convinced it was more than just another relationship.

As I pulled the key from my purse under the dim porch light, he drew me close, and we exchanged a long hug. Even in the pale light, the sadness on his face was visible as he whispered, "Good night, Annie," and walked away.

2 - Nightshades in Bloom

I turn on the lights and pour myself a glass of wine but put it aside. Alcohol could increase the headache intensity. My house needs cleaning. I put that aside, too. Instead, I call my dad. As a scientist, he always examines problems from several angles. I know he won't blame or judge. We've never kept any secrets from each other.

"Dad? I'm involved with someone..."

"Woman, criminal, or politician?"

"Worse. A man who lives overseas and--he's married."

"Well, you won't run into his wife at the supermarket."

"There's more... Um... His wife is a quadriplegic."

"Ooh, Annie! That's a lot to take on."

If I close my eyes, I can see his disapproving frown. The same reaction he gave me when I almost failed trigonometry.

"I hear your disapproval."

"I'm worried how it'll affect you. There is no happy ending to this situation."

"I've never felt this way about anyone. I've known him only for a month, but it's like he's always been part of my life." A pounding headache strikes and interrupts my train of thought.

"Annie? Are you there?"

"Still here. I know it's not ethical, but—"

"Ethics aside, this is a no-win situation. Are you willing to put yourself through so much?"

"I don't know. I'm still struggling with the whole 'cheating' thing."

"He's doing the cheating. He's the married one, not you."

"I'm participating!"

"What would you tell a patient with the same problem?"

"I'm asking myself the same question."

"I don't see what you'll gain from this relationship. A few weeks vacation?"

"I can't end it. It's like being pulled by a magnet. When I'm around him, I see only beauty in the world. At the same time, I feel silly falling so hard for someone I hardly know.

We haven't even kissed."

"Oh, boy..."

"What?"

"It's too late."

"I'm so confused. I'm like that moth circling a candle flame."

My father sighs into a long pause. "Love is not a choice. It's a storm that catches you by surprise. Just protect yourself. Don't change your life to fit his."

"I'm not moving to Argentina, if that's what you mean. Dad, can you please not tell Mom?"

"Annie—"

"I know. Just until I figure out what I'm doing, okay?"

We hang up with no solution, but we agreed to keep Mom in the dark. She lives in a black-and-white world. Aside from disappointment, it would hurt her to see me being the other woman.

After hours of stretching and curling in bed, wondering how many more lies I'll have to tell, I sit up and reach for my laptop. I search for a map of Argentina that displays all the provinces and regions. I know so little about South America in general. I trace a route between Virginia and Buenos Aires. Thousands of miles separate us, yet I feel closer to Daniel than I ever felt to Robert, the man I lived with for years. I browse through pictures of different locations, then zero in on Ushuaia, the southernmost city on the planet. Why is a land in Antarctica named Terra del Fuego?

I know so little about Daniel and the little I know is a warning to stay away. Yet, he awoke something in me I didn't know existed. Is passion more consuming when it's challenged? Is love more powerful when it's threatened? Or did I get manipulated into the situation?

It was so different with Robert. We've known each other since college. Our friendship made the transition to intimate roommates seamless. Yet, after two years of living together, Robert lost interest in sex and I was too tired to notice. Our schedules didn't leave room to wonder if it was love, friendship, or whatever. Before we figured out the "whatever", eight years drifted into the past.

Robert and I looked so good in pictures, people joked that our wedding photos would be in *Vogue*. He was my best friend, my confident, the rock I leaned on. I never worried about what he thought of my appearance. He rarely noticed what I wore or how I did my hair. Our strong bond provided a stable platform on which we built our careers. Our relationship was like postcards of old European castles: beautiful and solid on the outside, cold and empty inside.

One morning, we woke up like strangers on a train. We were down to finances by then: who kept Netflix, who got Amazon Prime, and who would change neighborhoods. We politely said goodbye and moved in different directions. Our love was strong enough for a parting with dignity but not big enough to grow yellow on pictures. As for *Vogue,* I never bought an issue anyway.

My churning thoughts precipitate into dehydration. Thirst and anxiety propel me out of bed, but I'm out of bottled water and my tap water has an aftertaste of copper. My choice is to enjoy the metallic flavor or suffer until morning.

/\ /\ /\

Daniel logs on with his phone. It's a beautiful day in Buenos Aires; a crowd of people behind him is shouting, laughing, and dancing.

"Buenas tardes, mi amor."

"Where are you?"

"I'm outside. Today is a great day for Argentina."

"Your soccer team won against Brazil?"

"Almost as good. Legislation just passed. Abortion is now legal. We've been fighting this battle for years. People are celebrating in the streets with music, dance... It's a huge party."

"Congratulations. I had no idea you were a feminist."

"I want my daughter to have a choice, you know? Give me two minutes and I'll re-login from my office."

When he logs in again, his hair is disheveled and his forehead glistens. I'm transported to our first meeting when he walked toward me with wet hair and a towel around his neck. My heart beats a little faster; I can see the movements on my chest—an advantage of big boobs.

"Can you talk while I chew on a few bites of this sandwich? I'm famished."

"I told my dad about us."

He lifts his chin and stops chewing. "Is that a good or a bad thing?"

"My dad is cool. It's my mother you have to worry about."

"I'm sorry. I'm putting you in a tough position. I hope you won't be at odds with your parents."

"Tell me about Tanya. What kind of teenager is she?"

"She's no trouble, except she likes to know where I am every minute of the day. If I have a business dinner, she doesn't go to bed until I come home."

"You're very close."

"It's more control than love, but I let her get away with it. She does so much to help her mother."

"She sounds well-adjusted."

"Most of the time, but she misses Nina the most when there is a school activity where the other kids come with their mothers."

"Can you attend these events with her?"

He reaches for a bottle of water and looks away. "I do, but it's not the same. It's easier now that she's older."

"Has she shown interest in boys yet?"

"Not that I know of. She doesn't socialize much. She's become a caregiver, but Nina developed a plan to enhance her education. She makes her read books, magazines, and poetry and they discuss them. Sometimes, the discussion turns into a heated debate."

"How clever!"

"She's more mature than most girls her age."

Talking about his daughter with so much love and admiration distances me from him. My face tightens as if splashed with ice water.

"Can I see more pictures of your family?"

Sensing my insecurities, he refuses. "Annie, you know what you're doing. You also know you shouldn't be doing it."

"Want my job? You won't like it. Pay's insulting." Sure, I know what I'm doing: obsessing over the woman who has the man I... love.

Many nights, I lie awake, wondering what his wife was like before "the Fall" as he calls it. She must be beautiful. Was she a good cook? A good lover? What special qualities does she possess to keep him loyal? It's an avalanche of questions to which I have no answers and, even if I did, would it end the anxiety or escalate it? Perhaps I should walk away. But I'm focused on what I want and purposefully ignore the obstacles ahead. How did I get caught in this game of love where desire is intensified when access is denied? This is the type of relationship I counsel patients against. *The Universe does have a sense of humor.*

Two days after our video date, a bouquet arrives at my office. The note says, "Love you tons, miss you miles. Daniel."

ΛΛΛ

I want to hear all about this Argentinian mafioso.
Hi, Tina.
Happy hour?
When?
2morrow. Have announcement.
Good news, bad news, or rumors?
Not rumors. 7 @ Dirty Martini?
K.

The bar is not crowded, but I would recognize Tina in a stadium during Super Bowl. She always wears gaudy colors and dresses according to the latest fashion trends on Instagram. While I'm down to Earth and reserved, Tina is exuberant, cheerful, and all-around hilarious.

"Annie!" she yells from the bar as soon as she sees me.

I approach her stool, and she hugs me without standing. "What's with the club soda?" I ask, surprised by the absence of her favorite cocktail—margarita.

"I've joined AA. That was my announcement."

"Yeah, one margarita a month. That's advanced alcoholism."

When Tina has something serious to discuss, she always starts with a joke. She calls it "warming up the audience". Judging by her shiny eyes and wide smile, she has some happy news to share.

"AA is where you can meet rich guys who've been dumped by their wives. They're ripe for the picking."

"Because they put all their money in the bottle."

"I said rich. Not proletarian."

"What happened to George?"

With her left hand, she swipes four fingers over her right ear to push her hair back and sparkles from a square diamond splash my eyes.

"No? You're getting married?"

"Yeah, but that's not the announcement? I'm four months pregnant."

"Honey, I'm so happy for you."

"We were planning on getting married next year, but this little brat is in a hurry. So, didn't want him to be born a bastard."

"I was planning on having a glass of champagne. I think I'll have two."

"Now, your Latin lover. I want to know everything."

Here goes my first lie. "Not much to tell yet. He lives in Buenos Aires. Very handsome, and he's crazy about me." I lock my lips on the glass of champagne while my eyes survey the wall of bottles behind the bar.

"What's wrong with him?"

I swallow more champagne. We've known each other for over a decade and we've never had secrets.

"What do you mean?"

"Why can't you look me in the eyes when talking about him?"

"It's new. It's COVID. He lives thousands of miles away. I don't think it'll go anywhere."

She put her hand on mine. "Nice, but I'm not your grandmother. Now, talk."

I put down the glass and face her. "He's married."

"But not impotent?"

I lower my voice. "I don't know! We never—"

"*That's* his problem."

"Didn't you hear what I said? He's married."

"If he's after you, he's not happy. Besides, the married ones are so grateful they can finally get laid. He'll shower you with gifts. I'm jealous. Pretty soon, I'll be married and pregnant." She laughs, exposing all her beautiful teeth. The couple next to us makes eye contact.

"Aren't you going to tell me to back off or something?"

She tilts her head and smiles. "His marriage is his problem, not yours. If he makes you happy, who knows?"

"I'm not a gambler."

"You can learn. Just avoid poker."

Tina deals with everything with laughter. Her motto is 'If you can't laugh, then make sure you're doing something more rewarding.'

Λ Λ Λ

The pain in my arm has given rise to severe headaches that don't resolve with medication. The last two nights, the pain drilled in my head like a jackhammer. When I woke up, my arm was numb. I text my friend and physician Don and ask for a referral to a neurologist.

As the elevator climbs the floors, the mirror reflects an image of a woman in perfect health. *Why am I here? It's probably some nerve thing. Worst case scenario, they'll tell me it's nothing.*

I adjust my mask when the doors open on the fourth floor and follow the signs to the Neurology & Chronic Pain Clinic. I arrive at an office with murals of what looks like Vivaldi's *Four Seasons* in print. One wall is a happy depiction of spring with pink dogwood blooms sprinkled on a crisp blue sky. Another wall expresses the joy of autumn with crimson foliage, golden yellow, orange, and purple leaves hanging from tall trees that line a long path leading nowhere. The rest of the space is filled with signs about masks and COVID symptoms.

A sweet receptionist named Ling checks me in. I lower my head for her to scan my forehead for a temperature reading.

"We received all your forms. I just need to scan your ID and insurance card."

"Are the doctors doing most of their consultations online?" I ask, pointing at the almost empty waiting room.

"A few. We still have a much lighter schedule than we used to. Lots of people are afraid to go to a doctor's office."

After Ling checks me in, I move to the waiting room. I sit next to a couple of women and an old man with a cane and shaking hands. Parkinson's. He drinks some water and struggles to put back his mask. I offer to help him, which he accepts with a warm smile. Behind the old man is a young woman, possibly in her twenties, accompanied by her mother. They're discussing Botox for headaches. My body relaxes into the seat. Maybe that's what I need. I'm developing chronic headaches.

A nurse comes out and calls my name. I follow her to an exam room where she checks my vitals. After she asks me a few questions about my general health, she escorts me to the doctor's office.

Dr. Dubeck greets me with a smile behind his two masks.

"What brings you in today?" he asks as he glances at the computer screen with my forms.

"I've been suffering from headaches for several weeks. The pain is debilitating and my arm is numb and tingly."

He removes his glasses and smoothes out his eyebrows. "How long have you been experiencing these headaches?"

"A few weeks. I ruled out food allergies by fasting for a couple of days and tried an elimination diet for two weeks."

"Is the pain all over or localized?"

"It's pressure, mainly in the back of the head, more toward the left. But it's really all over. It's like being hit with a hammer repeatedly."

"Any symptoms like nausea, blurred vision?"

"I felt like throwing up once. The pain was so bad, I had to lie down."

He lowers his white bushy eyebrows and mumbles something in his beard. His face reminds me of Mikhailovich Vasnetsov's painting *Savaoph, God the Father*. He hands me a prescription for a powerful headache medication and an MRI.

"Once the MRI is done, the results will come in the same day. My office will call you to schedule a follow-up visit."

No more lying or pretending. He clearly suspects a tumor and so have I—for weeks. I dial the radiology center from the waiting room to schedule the MRI. The earliest spot available is in three days. More time for the tumor to thrive.

On the drive home, I stop for a smoothie. I drink two gulps and my stomach locks. *A brain tumor. I have a brain tumor.* I keep repeating it out loud like a war announcement on a TV station. I stop on the side of the road to empty my stomach. The headache is now continuous. I wanted every cell in my body to prepare for the bad news, for a brutal treatment, for my life to turn upside down. Daniel. My parents. My patients. Friends. Silhouettes of people scroll before my eyes.

/\ /\ /\

The MRI results are in and I'm summoned to the neurologist's office. In the elevator, an older woman leans on a cane. Her uncombed wispy hair splashes the mirror of the elevator wall like a stain. Like a plant that blooms in the spring, bears fruit in the summer, withers in the fall, and dies in the winter, this old lady went full circle. I count the floors as the elevator beeps them. I know what they'll find. The question is, how advanced?

As soon as I sit down, the doctor pulls out stapled sheets of paper from a folder.

"Is anyone here with you?"

"No, just me."

If Daniel lived nearby, would he be here? I pretend he's sitting next to me and extend my hand on the chair.

"I'm afraid it's not good news."

"It's a tumor, isn't it?"

He examines my face with his piercing blue eyes. He purses his lips and nods. "The images show a tumor in the left hemisphere of the brain."

"What grade?"

"This type of tumor is called anaplastic astrocytoma. It develops from star-shaped brain cells called astrocytes. It's classified into four grades. Yours is grade three. It's fast-spreading and infiltrates surrounding tissues with tentacle-like structures, which makes complete excision difficult. If the tumor is not completely removed, it will grow back." He pauses to let me absorb the shock, then adds, "Fast."

"What's the prognosis?"

"First, you need surgery to remove as much of the tumor as possible. Then follow up with radiation and chemotherapy. With this treatment, twenty-seven percent of patients live five years post-diagnosis. But that's just statics."

"What are the side effects of surgery?"

"Some people have their speech impaired for a while; memory loss is common. But it's all temporary. With reeducation, many patients recover pretty well."

"And if I refuse radiation?"

"Nine months to two years."

We stare at each other. Then he leans back, exposing his large belly, opens the desk drawer, and hands me a business card.

"You have to meet with an oncologist. I suggest Dr. Drapeau at Suburban Hospital. We've already spoken. He has an opening for Monday afternoon."

On the way back to the car, I quell a few tears. A bed of pansies borders the sidewalk; their delicate petals flirt with the sun as the breeze sways them. They stare at me with their little black eyes. A chipmunk runs furtively to avoid me. I slow my pace to watch a couple of squirrels chase each other up a tree.

A car follows me to take my parking spot. The vast lot is full—so many altered lives. Many will improve, a few may even heal, but all will forever be defective. Soon, I'll be one of them: a patient. I'd like to cry, scream, cuss. But it's too late. One can't negotiate after the enemy has won. I need to live faster. I won't win the race, but I'll run as far as I can. The most arduous task is to prepare others. I don't know how to announce it to my father. How do you tell a father he'll lose a child who's not even forty? I don't have the words to express such news. He's not equipped to deal with such a loss.

I drive home mechanically. The doctor's grim face is imprinted on my mind. His voice echoes loud in my head: "*Cancer. Tumor.*" I speed through traffic and exit the highway.

I park the car, step out, and Ron waves at me. I wave back and hurry into the house. I open the door and put my purse on the console below the large picture of a girl walking on a beach with her hair flowing back. My father took the picture when I was twelve. Strange, how we always dream of big things, but happiness is made of small things

I spend the entire afternoon rehearsing my announcement. Trying to adjust to the new reality, I repeat several times, *"I have cancer."* I make a list of words to use to break the news to Daniel. How do I start? This isn't what a couple, newly in love, should discuss. English doesn't have a word that describes both anger and shame. But like a pregnancy, it can only be hidden for a while. Maybe it's the fear of losing him or the shame of being damaged, but I wish I could break it off and leave him with a beautiful memory. I don't want him to see me become... what I will become.

But there's a positive side: I'm no longer worried about Nina. Death will cancel my sin. I text Daniel before our usual Saturday phone call to ask for a video date. A computer screen is as close as we can get to a physical meeting. The intimacy of a face-to-face delivery somehow softens the blow.

I scour my closets in search of an outfit with vibrant colors. I settle on my lavender and white dress with little pink motifs that resemble birds in flight. Checking my appearance in the mirror brings up memories of our first date. His electrifying touch on my shoulder, our tête-a-tête dinner, and our only hug at my doorstep under the stars. Are these the only memories we'll ever share? I dab my wet eyes with a tissue before applying mascara. I fluff my hair and color my lips.

I set the laptop on the kitchen table with a basket of tangerines in the background. His face comes on the screen and his cheerful voice resonates through the Apples's sound system. "Hola, mi amor."

"Don't you look hot! Interesting tie?"

"Yeah, just got out of a meeting. Didn't have time to change. How are you?"

If I prolong the small talk, I may lose the courage. I have to do it fast, like spitting a bite of rotten fruit.

"Listen, I have some bad news. There is no way to sugarcoat it. I have a brain tumor."

Incredulous, he jerks his head back and stares at the camera, immobilized. "A brain tumor? What kind? What stage?"

"It's a very aggressive form of cancer. If they can't remove all of it, it will regrow."

His face is etched with questions and the pea that forms between his eyebrows when he's worried is now the size of a cherry. He lowers his eyes to the keyboard and sighs. We're both mute. Then comes the inevitable next question, which is nothing more than a code for "will you recover?".

"What's the prognosis?"

"If it grows back, less than two years, depending on its speed. If I go through the conventional treatment, possibly five years, but not more than that."

Like a lost traveler unsure which road to follow, we pause in search of appropriate words.

"There are other holistic nutrition-based therapies I'm investigating."

He's reassured by the glimmer of hope. His face relaxes. He lowers his shoulders and crosses his arms on the desk. "There is a clinic somewhere in northern Argentina. Can't remember the name now. A friend of mine's mother was treated there for stage-four liver cancer. She is now in remission."

"There are a few in California and Mexico, too, with good success rates."

"I want to come see you and discuss all this."

"There are COVID restrictions on travel."

"I'll find a way. Are you scared?"

"Not of death."

"I need to take care of a few things here and I'll be there as soon as I can."

My throat tightens. Does he feel sorry for me or is he attracted to defective women? "I-I don't think it's a good idea."

"Why not?"

"I don't want you to fly all the way from Argentina to see a sick person."

He tilts his head and moves closer to the camera and says in a counseling voice, "If we have only a few years, there is no time to waste. I wish I'd done more things with Nina before the Fall. But I was too busy building a career. I won't make the same mistake with you."

"But you can walk out of this one."

"Annie! Having cancer doesn't change my feelings for you. We were already planning to meet. If we wait until after your surgery, the borders might be closed by then. Lots of countries have banned travel until who knows when. There is also a risk they'll close the borders while I'm there."

I giggle. "We have a saying here: when it rains, it pours. I'd say it's a tornado."

He doesn't find my comment amusing. "Here is an idea. I can come just before surgery and stay a couple of weeks until you recover."

I shake my head and object. "Absolutely not!" Images of hospitals, tubes with dripping fluid, and needles crowd my mind. I blink hard to chase them away.

"It's settled then. I'll see you next week."

/\ /\ /\

September breeze shakes off more leaves from the sidewalk oak tree. They drift a while, delaying the fall, protesting death, then slowly descend to the ground, and gently give in to their fate. A line from one of Marvell's works echoes in my head. "But at my back I always hear / Time's wingèd chariot hurrying near."

When there is so little time left, people become voracious. They want to consume all of it to the last crumb. But how do you consume time? Do you enjoy it like ice cream, cold and fast, before it melts away? Do you sip it like wine, ever so slowly? Or pick through it like fruit, discarding rotten days? How do we stop the farmer Time from harvesting our days before they're ripe?

3 - Dim Light and Rhodochrosite

I empty my makeup case on the bathroom floor and compare eyeliners, concealers, lipsticks, blush. I try them one after another, wipe, reapply, wash, and start over. An hour passes before I'm pleased with the results. Clothes are already selected. I spent two days trying several outfits until I settled on a silver gray pantsuit with a short jacket and a pale red tank top. I check my appearance once more in the mirror, fluff my hair, and rub a few drops of Channel Mademoiselle on my neck. My body feels so hot and light, I could rise above ground. I jump in the car and wave at Ron. He raises a can of beer as I drive away.

On the way to the airport, I accelerate way above the speed limit. I lift my foot off the pedal at the sight of a police car.

The parking lot at Dulles Airport looks like a shopping mall on New Year's Day. COVID has its perks. I park close to the entrance and dash to the terminal.

After checking his flight status, I pace between the monitors and the rope barriers that hold the waiting crowds back from arriving travelers. I alternate between watching the clock, checking my cell phone, and staring at the monitors. Once his flight status changes from *"landed"* to *"in customs,"* I stand closer to the ropes. The black rubber doors open and close, spilling out people. Sometimes, a group emerges, then a couple looking lost, a single woman in a hurry, a family with a sleeping infant, followed by a crowd of young tourists rolling their suitcases. My heart skips each time the doors open. I peer past the travelers to locate him. It takes many heart leaps, many faces, and a seemingly month-long hour before his silhouette comes into focus. Our eyes lock and crinkle as we smile beneath our masks. I swoon.

It's all real. He's here. I remind myself to stop shaking, but a shiver runs over my skin.

"Welcome to Virginia," I murmur. We embrace with our masks on. We savor the moment, squeezing out all the gaps of the previous weeks.

He steps back, checks me up and down, then whispers in my hair, "You look smart."

At his suggestion, we booked a room in L'Auberge des Assassins, a French Bed and Breakfast in the Shenandoah Valley, about an hour from the airport. It's close enough to the city, but still isolated, with all the beauty of Virginia's countryside. Not a lot to do, but without crowds, an ideal spot during a pandemic.

Despite a sixteen-hour flight, he shows no sign of fatigue. He's as jovial as a child on his birthday. He sits comfortably in the passenger seat, head tilted back, legs stretched out, left arm leaning toward me. Perhaps the sexiest attribute of a man is confidence.

Somewhere past Manassas and before Marshall, he caresses my neck, sending electric tingles down my spine.

"I didn't sleep much on the plane."

What I couldn't tell him is I spent the night waiting for the day to rise. Instead, I smile and nod.

"So, how are you feeling? Any fatigue?" he asks.

"I want this time to be about us. I don't want to talk about anything sad."

"All right then. Let the vacation begin!"

He kisses my hand. His lips on my skin erase cancer from my mind.

"How did Tanya react to your leaving?"

"Jealous. She wanted to come. I've never gone on a vacation without her."

"Was she upset?"

"There will be other times."

I tighten my grip on the steering wheel and glance at him; we smile as to ascertain the veracity of the statement.

"She's at that age where she's starting to pay attention to fashion, makeup. Just a matter of time before she starts looking at boys."

"Did you take her shopping for her first bra yet?"

"Oh, no! My sister does the girl shopping with her."

We pull into the driveway of the Auberge. A heavy knot

coils in my stomach and my legs wobble when I exit the car. We retrieve our luggage from the trunk, ready to dive into our relationship, one-on-one, without video freeze, mute button, or disconnection.

At the reception desk, we're greeted by a young man with a shaved head, tattooed arms, and a beard. He gives us the key and wishes us a nice stay.

Daniel quips, "Do you think I'd look good with tattoos?"

"Only if you get a nose ring."

We step into a French provincial-style room with yellow floral curtains, pale-yellow speckled walls, and a large mahogany armoire against the back wall. A tall antique lamp stands behind a Louis XIII-style armchair facing the bed.

"How quaint!" he says.

He hangs his jacket while I fiddle with my cell phone to occupy my trembling hands. He removes his watch, gives me a reassuring glance as if we've done this before, and moves toward the bathroom with a pile of clothes.

"I'm going to shower and change." He's surveyed my mood, cataloged my emotions, and taken control.

I sit in the armchair with my arms crossed. The reality of his presence paralyzes me. I have an urge to leave or disappear.

He comes out of the bathroom, his hair still wet, pulled back. He's dressed in navy blue pants and a crisp white shirt. A thin belt hugs his waist. The style is reminiscent of 1950s Christian Dior. It's the kind of elegance that threatens other men and demands obedience from everyone else. I'm intimidated by his confidence and envious of his certainty.

He moves toward me. I feel crushed. He extends his arm above my head and opens the curtains.

"Why are you sitting in the dark? I want to see your face."

"Are you hungry? There isn't much around here. So, I brought snacks."

"Actually, I'm thirsty," he says as he sits on the bed to put on his shoes.

"Got you covered. Regular or bubbly?" I pull out two bottles of water from my bag. He chooses the San Pellegrino.

He eyes me to assess my readiness and declares, "OK, let's explore *Birginia* and grab a burger."

"Hey, I love burgers," I reply, a little more at ease.

"Me, too. With gooey cheddar cheese."

"I'll get you a veggie burger."

"Nah, I want the cholesterol. My arteries need to slow down."

The warmth of his laugh is soothing. His voice is soft but with volume, gentle yet firm. In person, I hear all the variations and nuances a computer sound system can't capture.

On the way to the car, we pause to admire the flowers bordering the path between the room and the parking lot. He snakes an arm around me and draws me close to him. "You're more beautiful than I remember." I rest my head on his shoulder and my anxiety slips away.

The sun shines brightly on this second Saturday in September. The leaves are still green, but the summer humidity has subsided. We drive to the surrounding towns. Antique stores line every street in rural Virginia. Some are filled with treasures, like Limoges plates, manual coffee mills, Depression glass vases, or collectible dolls. Others display an array of unusual objects ranging from painted toilet seats, Elvis beer glasses that read "*Thank you, thank you very much*," to perfume bottles with an eagle-head top. Other stores offer more useful memorabilia: music of the 70s, clothes from the 60s, baskets of vintage jewelry, and last-century phones all await a good home. Trash or treasure, here languishes America's rejected past, hoping for a fool to fall in love with it.

"There is a barrio in Buenos Aires called San Telmo. It has similar stores and a flea market every Sunday."

"I'm sure you have better stuff there."

"Same junk. But we don't have Elvis."

"You don't have Elvis?" I ask, feigning shock. "What kinda

country is that?"

He shrugs. "That's why Argentina is in turmoil."

"You gotta have Elvis. Our next trip is to Graceland."

He looks in the distance and nods. "Graceland. I'd like that."

We stop at several small towns: Lost Corner, Boyce, Briggs, and Berryville. Clark County is small but punctuated with a lot of hamlets with abandoned buildings. Mute witnesses to the progression of life, buildings that once were vibrant, filled with children's laughter, Halloween parties, and Christmas celebrations, turned into empty boxes of garbage, desecrated by time, forgotten by history. I wonder what life was like for those who occupied them. They had children, jobs, aspirations, and dreams. Did they ever make it? Did they leap into the future and leave the past behind, or did they go extinct like the passenger pigeon?

I slow the pace to comment on the landscape. "I find ruins fascinating. It's like a cemetery of a bygone era."

"Or a playground for the future. This is where they played until they grew up and moved to the next chapter of life."

I turn toward him. "That's one way to look at it."

He squeezes my hand and smiles. "My grandmother used to say, 'Every blooming flower is the birth of a seed.'"

I reply with a poem: "Thus, though we cannot make our sun/ Stand still, yet we will make him run."

"Lovely! Who's the author?"

"Andrew Marvell."

"You like poetry? I used to write poems when I was younger." He winks with a wry smile. "You're safe. They're in Spanish."

"They can't be that bad."

He chuckles. "Thankfully, nobody will ever find out."

In Berryville, we stop at Hip & Humble. The owner lifts his eyes from his newspaper to greet us, then continues reading. We enter a small room with a long dining table and a sidebar with pewter plates and random vintage objects. A large mechanical, monster-like sculpture made of wires stands in a corner. Its arms hang down like tentacles; its head is a wire ball with a large open mouth made of two metal plates. One webbed foot steps forward in a threatening gesture.

He notices my fascination with the art piece and moves closer, as if he wants to share this intimate moment between me and the sculpture. He rotates my shoulders to face him. I shiver. My heart is so full it expands to the limit of its surroundings, then a little more. My body softens like a creek after the ice has melted. There, inside Hip & Humble and before the monster, we kiss for the first time.

We leave the store holding hands; the rhythmic cadence of our steps echoes in my head like a church song. By the time we return to the car, the sun has dipped below the horizon and daylight is being swallowed by the approaching night. We drive back to the Auberge without conversation. Jet lag has finally caught up with him. He squints and opens his eyes to fight the gravity of heavy eyelids. The roads are empty, but I still obey the speed limit, which turns every little bump into a jolt.

We enter the room, close the door, and he immediately pulls me in for another kiss. This time deeper and longer, immersing me in a squishy cocoon.

I dig my fingers into his hair and murmur in his neck, "Why didn't you kiss me at the airport?"

"You were shaking."

"I'm sorry. It's not that I don't trust you, I—"

"You don't have to explain. Our relationship bloomed over a computer screen. It's uncomfortable when it becomes a reality, even a reality we want."

"Does this count as online dating?" I ask.

"No. I haven't asked you for money to bail out my construction crew in Ghana."

In the bathroom, I change and touch up my makeup before we head to dinner. When I come out, I find him stretched on the bed. I wait quietly in the armchair. A few minutes later, he opens his eyes, embarrassed; he sits up and adjusts the pillow behind his head. He checks my outfit—a short red dress with a décolleté that enhances a small pearl pendant.

"You look *sensacional!* Can we skip dinner?" he asks, gazing over my legs.

"And let that vegan menu go to waste? No way."

Probably expecting a salad and a fruit bowl, he raises an incredulous brow and smiles.

"Yes, I did call and asked them to prepare a menu for you."

He gestures for me to join him on the bed.

We lie next to each other, our body heat fusing and circulating freely while his hand pockets mine above his heart. A warm sensation stretches my body in his direction; he turns toward me for a kiss while holding me tighter. My entire being shrinks into a little fuzzy ball cradled in the safety of his touch.

"I think we need some champagne."

At the restaurant, a masked hostess greets us. Daniel asks for a corner table, away from traffic and voyeurs. But privacy is easy in a pandemic. The elegant dining room that used to seat many now has only three other tables with guests.

The hostess leads us near a window shielded by olive-green, goblet-pleated curtains. The table is adorned with heavy cutlery and large porcelain plates; the white tablecloth is divided by a runner that matches the wallpaper—a pale-pink background with delicate purple and white flowers. The decor reminds the guests of summer in the French countryside and serves as a base to hold the overflowing romantic aura.

The elegance of the table, the beauty of the room, and the soft light dripping from the sconces like honey create a dream-like atmosphere that conjures up happiness. I drink it all and a wave of joy sweeps away the gloom of the last few days.

Shortly after we sit down, a bottle of champagne arrives in a silver-plated bucket on top of a tall stand the waitress sets next to him. As protocol dictates, she presents the label to the person who placed the order. Their interaction tickles my pride. Looking only at him, the waitress rotates her body slightly toward him and tilts her head in the opposite direction, exposing her beautiful neck and a Hollywood smile. She pours him a small amount to taste and continues to describe the champagne—notes of peach, not too sweet, with a pear finish. Without even a glance my way, she asks him where he's from and how long he's staying in town.

"We're here for a few days." He nods at me. "She's my Virginia tour guide."

Our eyes meet. She blushes, fills our flutes, and leaves. What went through her mind was probably "What a lucky woman!" What went through mine was "Why am I given such a beautiful gift with an expiration date?"

We lift our glasses to commemorate the moment. "What should we drink to?" I ask.

"To defeat," he solemnly says, lifting his chin to dominate the scenery.

"That's a rather strange endeavor."

"To defeating cancer." He leans over and kisses me.

I'm not sure which one provoked the most uplifting sensation, the kiss or the champagne, but cancer is no longer on my mind.

"So, what's with the name Lorenzo? Isn't that Italian?"

"It's a Spanish name meaning 'from where the laurel trees grow'. Quite common in Argentina as a last name. In Italy, it's a first name, I believe. How about you? Have you ever been curious about your biological parents?"

"I'm happy with my adoptive parents. They did so much for me. There is nothing I could do my father wouldn't understand or forgive. My mother is a little strange, but still a good mother."

"Strange? How so?" He pours more champagne into my flute. "Well… she doesn't know how to express emotions.

When I was little, if I fell and cried, she'd yell at me instead of hugging or kissing me."

"How interesting!"

"That's just how she is. My dad is more affectionate. I'm closer to him."

"I'd like to meet them someday."

That hit me like a punch in the face. We may never meet each other's families. We may never become a family. With the back of my hand, I move a few locks of hair from my face to distract from the gloomy thoughts that just punched me. Then I get hold of myself. I cannot afford to waste this beautiful evening. I lift my glass and put on my best sultry pose and proclaim, "I want to drink to serendipity."

The waitress returns to check on us, but we haven't opened the menus yet. I'm not hungry. All the usual sensations, such as hunger, thirst, and fatigue, have been replaced with yearning, anticipation, and bouts of panic. Being with someone so magnetic who stirs my entire being is a new experience. No wonder they call it *falling* in love. In my case, it's *flying* in love. I'll run out of time before the fall.

The menu takes vegan gastronomy to a new level: velouté de butternut squash with ginger espuma, beet carpaccio on a bed of microgreens, plant-based king crabs with braised Belgian endives on a sunchoke divan, Seitan steak au jus, consommé forestière with roasted cauliflower and bacon bits—certified plant-based.

I say, "I did not know vegans had haute cuisine."

"Anything you can do with meat, you can do better with plants, my dear."

After the meal, we walk back to our room, holding hands. Once inside, he gently pulls me toward him for a long hug. I wrap my arms around his neck and feel his chest against my breasts. Many sensations interweave inside me like threads in a loom, moving at the beat of a paddle. He pulls away and walks toward his bag.

"I have something for you." He produces a small pink suede box and hands it to me. "It's something you've never seen before."

An oval-shaped glossy, creamy pink gemstone lay on a plush white fabric. It's about two inches long and hangs from a white gold chain, held by a delicate two-pronged bail. It's clearly been handmade by someone who has the patience of an artist and the love of an artisan.

"A pink gemstone? Looks like candy."

"It's one of a kind."He drapes it around my neck and guides us to sit on the bed.

"Rhodochrosite. It's the national gemstone of Argentina. The best specimens are found in the northwestern part of the country. You see the white lines? That's what makes it special. If the stone is too pink, without flaws, it's not as elegant."

"Gorgeous. Some scientific studies actually confirmed that pink is a mood-enhancing color."

"It's also the color of hope," he says, a twinkle in his eyes.

Inside the box, a little card lined with vellum is engraved with the name of the designer, a woman who's been making jewelry for decades under the guidance of spirits.

"She said she works only by inspiration and when instructed by her guides. Whatever that means."

I read aloud the English version of the message this jeweler wanted to communicate to the world.

"Rhodochrosite promotes self-healing, self-love, and inner happiness. Its pink color directs your energy toward emotional healing. It supports recovery from past trauma, or past lives that have not been healed yet."

He laughs. "I wanted to make sure you're cleansed of all past lives."

"I'm out of a job. If this precious stone can heal my patients from trauma, it's more affordable than a shrink."

"Imagine the money they'll be saving in the next life!" He chuckles, then turns stoic. "When you wear it, you'll feel my presence."

"You put a chip in it to track my whereabouts?"

"And a camera."

We slowly fall on the bed and he covers me with his body. Words are lost in kisses. Clothes slowly come off. We discover each other under the dim light of an antique lamp. There are no more questions, no more anxiety, just soft, incandescent gestures of love. Ever present under his exploring hands, my insecurities surrender to serenity. I enter a new dimension where fear and cancer no longer exist.

His soft voice wraps around me like a fluffy blanket. Love is a different breed of happiness. The kind one drinks slowly, and like alcohol, it goes quickly to the brain. I'm drunk with happiness. I rest my head on his chest and play with the few hairs standing on his skin. I don't want to fall asleep. I don't want the night to end.

The morning comes way too soon, with the sun shining through the yellow curtains. Without opening his eyes, he scoops me up and cradles me in his arms, my head under his chin. His hand runs over my back and I'm submerged in a sea of tranquility. My defenses thawed and melted away, new sensations awaken parts of my body that were, until now, dormant. Like a wilted plant receiving water and sunshine, I become more alive—vibrant. Swirling colors dance all around me like psychedelic art. Each movement, each breath, each kiss lifts me higher into that diaphanous cloud. I savor every second with gusto, for these delectable moments may be all I'll ever know. At thirty-eight, I experience the transformation of a young girl entering adulthood.

Energized by lovemaking, I feel an urge to talk. I comment on the beauty of the garden and the different flowers. I flip through the brochures and select things to do during our stay in town. We talk in the bedroom, we talk all the way to the breakfast room, and we talk more between each waiter's interruption. Our conversation flows naturally with synchronicity. We have bridged the gap between online fantasy and reality.

The breakfast room is smaller than the dining room and features the Alsace region. Jean-Marc, the owner, designed each dining room to reflect a different region of France. A large painting of the Strasbourg Cathedral with its renowned astronomical clock drapes the facing wall. The ceiling—the only dark accent in the room—is lined with mahogany beams. Bright colors of muted yellow walls, red curtains, and blue china give the room a cheery vibe.

The waiter brings our beverages and asks if we're ready to order. Daniel gestures for me to go first.

I forgo the bacon and eggs and opt for a vegan breakfast. "Loaded oatmeal, please."

"Loaded oatmeal for me and sweet potato muffins."

After the waiter leaves, he bows his head and says softly, "You don't have to change your diet on my account."

"Actually, the loaded oatmeal sounds intriguing and I can't resist toasted almond flakes and cinnamon."

He pours soy milk into his coffee cup; he takes it to his lips, then sets it back down.

"Too hot?" I ask.

His eyes wander on the table before facing me. "When's the surgery?"

"Two weeks from Tuesday." I turn my face and cast my gaze on the beautiful garden waking up beyond the windowpane. The flowers are slowly opening their petals to the sun.

"Have you told your parents yet?"

I've forgotten about cancer and resent the reminder. I lift my shoulders and shake my head. "Don't know how."

"I need a contact number for when you're in the hospital. Someone I could call if I don't hear from you."

I reluctantly give him my father's number since I don't intend to tell many people. Cancer is an intimate conversation that makes me feel angry and ashamed— the kind of shame felt by rape victims. In a matter of days, I went from an accomplished professional to a rotting cancer wreck. He's so together and perfect and I'm damaged, about to be discarded. I excuse myself to go to the bathroom before he notices my discomposure. I wet my hands and pump soap on them. I knead the lather until it forms a silky white paste, then run the water and watch it slip away as I stare at the mirror. Under the shadow of doom, my face still glows.

Back at the table, I lower my head and my face undulates in the cup of tea; I swallow a mouthful as to warm up my voice. "There's... huh... there's something you need to know." My voice quits.

"What is it?" He holds my hand between his palms.

I swallow more tea. "Brain surgery may cause a personality change."

"What kind of change? You'll forget about us?"

"Not exactly. I may become more aggressive, depressed, or agitated. It's impossible to predict, but the change is within three months of the surgery and usually short-lived." I choke back tears. "I'll send you some literature."

The ceiling has dropped a few inches lower. The dining room has become small and suffocating. He signs the bill, then lifts his head to face me.

"Is that all?" he asks.

The corners of my mouth move into an involuntary smile. "Well, yes. Maybe." I turn my head to the door to watch the waiter walk toward our table.

"Would you like more tea or coffee?"

"No, thank you." Daniel hands him the signed bill.

"So, what else are we to expect?"

Damn! My cheeks heat up. "Some people become sexually overactive."

"You'll have to move to Argentina." He holds my hand and we laugh in earnest.

Λ Λ Λ

Two, three, four, then the final fifth day, all quickly swallowed by time and swept into the past. Several times, I was seized by panic at his approaching departure. It's a demarcation between real life and a universe filled with treatments, pain, and devastation. But cradled in our love, it was easy to push those thoughts away. I want him to remember me with positive and joyful notes. Cancer shouldn't be part of our time together—as short as it may be. I cannot wish it away, but I won't honor it or let it steal my joy.

Gone are the Indian summer days. Virginia weather can change abruptly from summer to winter in a matter of hours. We drive to the airport under drumming rain and dark sky, to the beat of slashing windshield wipers.

He holds my hand during the entire trip and throws a few smiles my way whenever I glance in his direction. A form of incomplete reassurance that leaves me yearning. The pandemic, the upcoming medical "mistreatments", and the distance will make it difficult for us to reunite again. Life has gone from complicated to a convoluted web of thorny knots.

"I'm sure the procedure will go well. I wish I could be there with you."

My left hand squeezes the wheel and my jaw tenses. I'm sure he can see my eyebrows drawing closer. "I don't want anybody to see me in a hospital bed."

He kisses my hand and smiles. "I'm not anybody." He sighs. "It could be months before we meet again." He pauses and stares in the distance; his jade-green eyes shine with little gold threads. "This has been the best vacation I've had in years. Thank you."

Then comes the airport separation. He holds me tight and I refuse to let go until I'm startled by a woman bumping into me. He cups my face in his hands and kisses me. "You'll be okay. I love you." The escalator swallows his silhouette and carries him away from me.

My legs are numb; my mind empty; the opposite escalator descends me to the exit. I feel gutted. I'm in no hurry to return to the crushing emptiness at home. I sit on a bench to regain my composure. I cross my wrists on my mid-section to squeeze out the hollowness and rest my head on my knees. A cleaning lady stands next to me with a broom and toxic cleaning gear. "Ajou okay, mam"? I lift my head and nod. The phone rings.

"Cara, I'm about to board the plane. I'll see you soon, okay? Love you." Like a gentle summer rain, his voice washes over me and softens the cold edges of my body.

To dispel the oppressive silence on the drive back, I increase the volume of the CD player to full blast and let Eric Clapton cry for me. Traffic is no longer an issue on the highway. I drive robotically, making instinctive wheel adjustments and ignoring the surrounding details of the road.

It's early evening when I reach my gated neighborhood. The median is bare; its dirt stirred where they cut down the Sun Goddess. Her little carcass, broken into pieces, rests on the sidewalk. It decorated the front of the block for years. It enchanted everyone with its vibrant yellow and fragrant roses. After it became infected with some disease, its leaves turned brown, its little trunk and branches dried up and became brittle. Now, it lies on the sidewalk like ordinary trash.

Ron is taking his beer for a walk. "Did you go on vacation, dear? Haven't seen you in a few days." He walks toward me, unmasked.

"I went on a little retreat."

"Good. Nobody does anything fun anymore. I put your mail in the basket on the back porch. Didn't want it to pile up in the front."

"Thanks, Ron. I'll get you some beer."

"You're welcome, sweetheart."

I enter the house and curl into a ball on the couch. A text message from Tina pulls me out of my Weltschmerz.

R u abducted by aliens?

Only been a week.

Dinner? Guesswhat im Craving?

Ice cream?

Fried onion rings.

W or without sour cream?

Honestly, i wake up middle of nt to eat'm. George thinks i shouldn't go out.

I think he's rt. You have to protect ur baby.

It's time to spread the news. I clear my throat and ask to use FaceTime.

"Tina, I need to tell you something." I pause and straighten my back. "I don't want you to freak out, okay?"

"You're getting married?"

"No."

"Sounds serious."

"I have a brain tumor."

Her eyes immediately fill with tears as she releases a piercing shrill. "How could you do this to me?"

"To you?"

"I want my best friend to enjoy this pregnancy with me."

"I will. They'll remove the tumor and I'll be fine. But we won't be seeing each other for a while."

"Oh, it's benign?"

"We'll know more after the surgery. A lot of people have tumors. Once they get them removed, they're fine. I don't want you to worry, okay?"

"When's the surgery?"

"Next week. The hospital allows only two visitors and my parents are coming. But you can visit after I come home."

Tears run down her cheeks, but she still wants to laugh. "Oh, Annie, it's so unfair. Is it because you're too smart and your brain is expanding?"

We laugh out loud for several minutes. "Absolutely. My brain needs more room. I now have to learn Spanish."

She mewls. "Take care of yourself, okay? And holler if you need anything."

"I will."

"Love you."

"Love you, too."

I review the schedule for the upcoming days: PCR test tomorrow, followed by a pre-op meeting with the doctor. I check where I need to be and when and ignore all other details. The night has fallen; the house goes dark after I close the laptop. It's too early to go to sleep but too late to do anything. I sit in the dark and let the memories of the last few days fill my mind and uplift my spirits.

4 - Harvesting Tentacles

Mid-afternoon, I finally get the motivation to open my travel bag. I toss the clothes in the laundry basket and hug the necklace Daniel gave me. A heavy weight in my mid-section pulls me down. I sit back on the couch and tears stream down my face.

Daniel's departure yesterday left me hollow. I floated between hope and despair until I fell asleep. I haven't yet mastered the courage to call my parents. The phone is a lever controlling the blade of a guillotine. I've been staring at the clock most of the afternoon to determine the best time to call them and deliver the blow.

I procrastinate until 8:00 p.m. in Oregon.

"Mom? Is Dad with you?"

"He's in his study."

"Can you please get him? I need to talk to both of you."

"We're both here and you're on speaker. Is everything okay?"

Despite her inability to articulate human emotions, my mother has a maternal instinct that could find me in a jungle. I clench my jaw, then swallow. I stall.

"Annie? What's wrong?" she asks.

"I… I have a brain tumor."

"What… What? How?" she says, her voice shrill. "When did… How long have you known? How big is the tumor?"

"They think it's in the early stages. I'm getting surgery next week."

"Did you get a second opinion?" My mother's cascade of questions is a mask for the shock. I've been translating her emotions since childhood.

With a shaky voice, my father interrupts. "Where in the brain is the tumor located and what's the prognosis?"

"It's in the left hemisphere."

The silence that follows is anything but gold; it's a thick, sticky mud that smears seconds into eons. Hearing the anguish in his voice scissors through my insides.

"The treatment consists of surgical removal, radiation, and chemo. It seems small enough that the chances of removing most of it are still good."

"What's the survival rate after treatment?" he asks.

I give them the background information such as the type of tumor, its ramifications, and different treatments, but my mother cuts to the chase.

"Annie? You haven't answered the question."

The line goes silent again. I'm in no hurry to shatter their hopes. When I finally find my voice, I distort the truth the best I can, but my mother can read between the different tones of my voice. Though she first laid eyes on me when I was three weeks old, her maternal instincts have been just as strong as I imagine any birth mother's would be.

"We'll know more after surgery."

"We need a second opinion," she insists.

"The MRI doesn't lie, Mom."

It takes several tries to convince her a second opinion isn't necessary.

"Give me your surgery date, and we'll be there."

"You don't have to do that, Mom. Tina and Robert can take care of anything I need. Besides, I can get necessities online. There are organizations that deliver food and groceries."

"We'll be there during surgery and I'll stay a few days after your release."

Before we hang up, in unison with my father, my mother says, "I love you." That's more shocking than the cancer diagnosis. She's experiencing a personality change before I do. I've never heard her say these three little words.

All my life, my mother has never been overly emotional. When I hugged her, she turned into a statue—not the smooth, fragile marble ones found in museums, but the solid, craggy cement ones used to decorate gardens. I've never seen my mother hug anyone except the dog. When Fred climbed her legs, tongue out, nose up, tail wagging, she put her arms around him, lowered her head to receive the kisses, and turned into a ball of cotton candy.

When I went to college, my mother did suffer from

separation anxiety. She called regularly and her way of saying she missed me was through questions about my well-being. She would first ask if I'd done my laundry, if I'd gotten enough sleep, or if there were any topics I was struggling with. As soon as I confided that I was tired or skipped meals, she'd raise her voice to tell me to make better decisions. But it was easy to discern her angry voice—a stream of words punctuated with *don't*—and her "I love you" voice, which was soft and laced with warmth.

There are no words to comfort them. Nothing would change reality; phrasing things softly cannot reduce the shock when a parent hears her child has cancer.

Monday evening is my last video date with Daniel. Who knows how long after the surgery I'll be able to show my face before the camera? To make the event special, we decided to have a virtual dinner together. I bought a frozen vegan pizza and threw it in the oven.

He logs on with a plate of lasagna on the desk.

"That lasagna better be vegan."

"A friend of mine has a vegan restaurant. I stopped by this afternoon."

We take turns eating and talking.

"A lot of people undergo brain surgery and completely recover," he says with a hopeful tone and a small frown.

"I know…" I swallow a bite of pizza."If only the president would get one!"

"He needs a brain transplant."

"They told me I should be up and running in about two to three days but probably not ready for video."

"I wish I could be there with you, but there are no flights from here to DC."

"I'll be fine. My parents will be there."

"I know. Still frustrating to be so far away."

"It makes for a better story. All my friends are envious that I'm seeing someone from Buenos Aires."

"It's a unique city in South America. Can't wait to show you around."

My body stiffens as if I just received an ice shower. This could be our last conversation with all my faculties. I repress those thoughts. "As soon as I feel better, I'll come visit."

We end the video with his usual "love you tons, miss you miles." We project ourselves into the future to minimize the impact, but we both know brain surgery is an invasive procedure with uncertain outcomes.

ΛΛΛ

"Where's Fred?" I hear myself mumble.

"Honey? You're awake. How're you feeling?" My eyes are still closed, but I recognize my father's voice.

"Like a truck drove over me. I just saw Fred walk out. Can you catch him?"

"Do you want some water?"

"No, just find Fred."

I wake up after what I thought was hours of sleep, but the wall clock indicates only thirty minutes have passed. My parents' silhouettes appear in a fog. I slowly open one eye while the other remains shut. Wires drop from my head to meet more wires attached to my hand. More wires on my chest are hooked to a monitor. I murmur something that my mother understands as "cold," so she covers me with blankets. My father sits next to me with his usual calm. Occasionally, they whisper something to each other. I want to ask for water, but my throat is dry and my voice is gone. I drift back into sleep.

The surgeon wakes me. His face is stoic, but he cracks a forced smile. "How are you feeling?"

"Is my brain clean now?"

He's caught by surprise. "Funny. Glad you're in high spirits. Your surgery went well."

He approaches to examine his work and continues talking, his voice thumping in my head like a sledgehammer. The nurse asks me to give her a pain grade between one and ten. I tell her fifteen. She takes a syringe and injects one of the ports in the IV line. A few minutes later, the pain is gone.

The surgeon talks to my parents while I doze off.

At 8:00 p.m., my parents, have left. The lights are now dim; the door is ajar, making me a spectator to the activities of the night staff. Traffic in the hallway is constant; all the sounds are amplified and feel close to my head. Between the nurses running back and forth, the techs moving equipment, and the patients moaning their woes, it's like a Fourth of July parade gone wrong. I eventually ignore the noise and the lights and drift into what is more unconsciousness than sleep.

I wake up thinking it's morning, but the clock reads 3:00 a.m. The boredom makes falling back to sleep arduous, so I let my imagination wander to relive the first time I met Daniel on the scuba diving boat. I glide through the water behind him, surrounded by schools of vibrantly colored fish. I follow him through cliffs of coral and sea vegetation. We look at an eel and other sea creatures hiding under stones or in holes. I feel his comforting presence like a bowl of ice cream after a disappointing meal. Then all thoughts stop and I blackout.

A hospital is not a restful place. It's where the damaged and defective are handled. A nurse wakes me up at daybreak to take my vitals. My sleep is disrupted, I turn on the television. My heart jumps out of my chest when I see a movie with Thorsten Kaye. It's as if he and Daniel were twin brothers. Same hair, same thick eyebrows, and same pride in the eyes. I want to hug the screen.

My parents arrive before breakfast and I'm happy to see them. My father has a big smile on his face and reminds me the surgery went without a glitch. I'll just have a puffy eye for a while. My mother looks more worried as she hurries to fluff the pillow behind my head and helps me sit up before she presents me with the breakfast tray. I'm not hungry, but the omelet looks appetizing. I nibble on it, then push it aside and reach for the mug of tea.

Layers of tape cover the IV portal on the back of my left

hand. A bag of fluid hangs above my head. I check the bandages, crowning my head. My father studies my movements with a serious face.

"I'm going to tell that story to your boyfriend."

"What story?" I lift my shoulders to shift positions, though doing so sends sharp spears of pain through my head.

"When you woke up from surgery, the first thing you remembered was a dog who died decades ago."

"Oh, yeah. Fred was my baby."

"I remember. You became a mom at six years old until he grew bigger than you."

"I still miss him." Tears run from the corner of my eye, wetting the pillow. In the absence of a sibling, Fred was my twin. We did everything together, including sleeping in the same bed. "Did they remove the tumor completely?"

The answer is a long time in coming. My father breaks the silence.

"Alas no. They removed all its tentacles, which were superficial, but the tumor itself is rooted a little deeper, so there is still a small amount left. He said it can be shrunk or completely eradicated with radiation therapy."

I now understand what people feel when they learn their plane is about to crash.

My father hands me my cell phone. "It's been beeping all morning. Will you tell the poor guy you're OK?"

I open WhatsApp to find five waiting messages. He's already online and, as soon as my status changes to online, he starts typing. My mind numbs the pain, deletes the hospital scene, and transports me into a peaceful bubble for the two of us.

Cara, how are you?

OK. Was totally out of it ystrday but lil btr this am.

Can I call you?

In a couple of hrs. My parents r here and I'll get a lot of visits from doctors n nurses shortly.

I'll call you at noon, Your time. Get some rest.

K, love you.

Te amo.

My parents relate anecdotes about their work, people we know, and the latest outrageous comments by the President of the United States. I listen, smile, and nod to reassure them I'm awake. A nurse comes in and hands me a new mask.

At noon on the dot, Daniel is on the phone. My parents leave the room to give us privacy.

"Did the surgery go well?"

"Very well."

"Are you in pain?"

"Just a headache, but they gave me meds. I'm feeling good. Just tired and creeped out by all the wires hanging from my hand and my chest."

"Can you move?"

"Yep. Oh, got a free hairstyle, too. It's fetching."

He takes a moment before responding. "I'm sure you look gorgeous. If I lived closer, I would've been there by now to cover you with kisses."

"I don't want you to see me until my hair grows back."

"Argentina just closed its borders, so I'm not sure when we'll see each other again."

"Good timing, Argentina. By the time we meet, I'll be as good as new."

"When do you go home?"

"In a couple of days."

Then he chokes with tears.

"I'm fine. Once I get out of here, everything will go back to normal..." E*ventually*.

"I know. I just wish there was something I could do."

"There is. Send me pictures of Buenos Aires. I want to see you dance tango."

"You're bad."

"But you like it when I'm bad."

The nurse comes in with a lunch tray, though my appetite is still absent. After she leaves, I push the platter aside and sob. I'm not supposed to be here. There is so much life in me. There is so much I want to experience. My father-holds me while my mother insists I eat.

/\ /\ /\

I leave the hospital with a long prescription for daily pills and a list of therapists—physical, mental, the works. As we enter the house, I head straight to the couch. My body has turned into Jell-O: no bones, no cartilage, just a soft heavy blob. I close my eyes, but I'm way too tired to fall asleep. The mind is engaged in a tug of war with the body: the latter wants to sink into darkness and rest; the former wants to live every minute. It's an aggravating dichotomy I can't control.

My mother keeps asking if I want to drink or eat. She fluffs my pillow, covers me with a blanket, and tries, using all the ways she can, to say "I love you" without words. Another sign she's hurting; I have no words to comfort her. My dad keeps telling her to leave me alone so I can get some rest. We smile at each other.

/\ /\ /\

Two weeks after surgery, my parents drive me to the neurologist. The incisions are healing without complications. Soon, my hair will grow back. There is no prognosis as to my other symptoms. Headaches, black holes in memory, and poor balance are all part of the pathology, he says. They will resolve at an unknown time.

"If I pursue the traditional treatment, what are the side effects?"

He turns to the drawer behind him, grabs a brochure, and puts it in my hands.

"There are short-term and long-term side effects. During treatment, some patients experience headaches, extreme fatigue, hair loss, and burns at the treatment site. In the long term, there is a risk of memory loss, maybe vision and hearing problems. The brochure will give you a complete list of symptoms, including the rare ones."

"I will not seek treatment."

He purses his lips, lowers his head, and stares at his withered fingers curled into a ball on the desk, then lifts his droopy eyes.

"Without treatment, the tumor will most certainly grow back."

"Based on what I learned from various scientific papers, with treatment, I can also get other tumors or a stroke."

"But that's rare."

"I could be the lucky one percent mentioned in this brochure."

He dismisses my questions about different treatments that don't involve radiation and advises me to stay on the anti-seizure medication—for an unknown *while*. There are no answers, no recovery path, and no hope. The only certainty is the regrowth of the tumor. The remaining root will seek revenge and grow even faster than before. Radiation therapy doesn't guarantee a cure, only a delay of the inevitable; but it does guarantee brain damage. I could lose my memory and will struggle to find my words; learning anything new might require a massive effort. Not to mention damage to hair follicles, resulting in wispy, fuzzy hair.

Refusing treatment is a death sentence; treatment is a path to destruction. Either way, statistics are clear, my chances of surviving beyond five years are slim to none. My teeth grind; I squeeze my hands into fists; my rage implodes. *NO! I can't accept that!*

ΛΛΛ

After my parents leave, I open the laptop to watch my pre-cancer life slip away. Work schedule, plans for the future, and the pictures I took with Daniel. I pause. Linger. Then I open the browser and sift through scientific articles to gain insight on what happens after the brain has been altered. After pages of monotonous repetition of what I already know, the conclusion is unanimous: conventional treatments only extend life by a few months or up to five years. Depending on the level of radiation therapy, damage to the brain might be irreversible.

I lie on the couch, watching hours and days drain from my life. I transferred all my patients to my colleague, Tom. My only communication is with Daniel, during which I often struggle to find my words. Whenever I experience a black hole, the functioning part of my brain randomly picks another word to compensate. In our last conversation, I wanted to ask him about his daughter. Instead, I asked about his mother.

One of the side effects of brain surgery is mood swings, due to the trauma to the brain. I keep my conversations short and infrequent. Thinking about Daniel only fills me with shame and rage. I have entered a new world where the altered and damaged live. The final phase of life, where the only occupation is waiting for the deterioration to complete.

Like a cat, my window is my television. I watch people go to work, walk their dogs, or push strollers. I so wish I could smoke or drink. The crushing fatigue keeps me horizontal. Food is delivery; clothes are pajamas. No need for a shower or makeup.

I keep a rigid schedule. I alternate between YouTube videos, sleeping, and feeling enraged. It's not the kind of anger that makes one yell or break things. It's a rage that seethes and explodes like a volcano. In six to nine months, I will turn into an idiot who doesn't recognize anyone; I'll slobber and talk in word salad. It's a slow death without awareness or dignity. I want to smash this head against the wall to speed up the process. I want it burned and thrown into a common dumpster. No ashes spread in the ocean or on mountains. Trash doesn't deserve to be honored. The phone rings. I'm too angry to ignore it.

"Hola, mi amor! How are you feeling today?"

He's always annoyingly cheerful, so I hide my rage. I respond with a terse "Fine." A word that's nothing but a euphemism for "I'm pissed off." The line goes silent for a second. Then I proceed with the axe.

"Listen, I don't think we should be in touch anymore. I want you to move on and be happy." More silence follows.

"I think that's my decision to make."

"You want to watch me disintegrate?" The tone of my voice rises uncontrollably.

"Annie? You can't talk to me like that." His usual commanding voice is coated with a soft sadness. It's no use. I can't hear him anymore.

"Then stop calling me!"

"Cara, you need help."

"Go to hell!"

I throw the phone. It hits the wall, leaving behind a crack in the drywall. I fold my knees and curl into a ball. Then, an unexpected dread seizes my lungs. The idea of never talking to him again suddenly sinks in and a sharp pain pierces my belly. *It's for the best,* I lie to myself. I so want to cry, but nothing comes out, just a sharp pain that keeps digging inside of me. Paradoxically, I don't want it to stop. For the first time in weeks, I don't care about cancer. I have a bigger loss to nurture.

The phone rings. I doze off and let it go to voicemail. It rings an hour later and wakes me up. I glance at the screen.

"Yes, Dad."

"Annie? Are you OK?"

"I'm fine." My patience has expired and I have no words to waste.

"You don't sound fine."

"Why are you calling, exactly?"

"Because I'm your father and I'm worried about you."

His voice is soft and cuddly. He doesn't deserve such a rude response; I get hold of myself and apologize.

"Mom got a ticket. She'll be there tomorrow."

"Is that a threat? I really don't need anyone yelling at me right now."

"We both want to help you recover. I'm in the middle of

exams. I can't break free at the moment."

When I was a child, whenever I was upset, my father's soft voice and warm hugs made the world a happy place again. Today, he uses the same voice to comfort me. Far from feeling better, but my rage is transformed into melancholy.

ΛΛΛ

Mid-afternoon. I'm still in pajamas when my mother knocks at the door. I have to brace myself for translation—criticism means affection. Her method for showing love is to reprimand, make a to-do list, and force-feed me.

We exchange an awkward hug. "Hi, Mom. You didn't need to come all this way."

She stands in the living room, and before she puts her suitcase down, she delivers her ghastly survey. "When was the last time you cleaned this place?"

"Don't know. Why?"

"Annie? Your house is in shambles! You've been living like this for five weeks?"

"Well, cancer doesn't afford me the luxury to worry about interior decorating."

As I lie back down on the couch, my mother gets to work. She picks up pizza boxes, Chinese carry-out boxes, tea mugs, paper plates, used napkins, and clothes scattered around the living room. She empties the fridge of old leftovers, cleans the kitchen sink, and then sits next to me.

She puts a hand on my forehead and sweeps my hair back. "Honey, will you let me run you a bath?"

"Are we expecting company?"

She smiles. "You smell bad." Brutal honesty is another way my mother shows love. "Come on, I have mango shower gel. It smells like ice cream." We both laugh and she helps me stand.

ΛΛΛ

With my eyes closed, I relish in the soothing fluidity of warm water on my skin. My back against the bath pillow, I stretch my legs in the bathtub. Then, like a storm that breaks without warning, my mind pivots to him. I get lost in a whirlwind of questions: What would our life be like if we could be together? Would we have children? Would we travel? I project myself into a time and space where all is possible. It smooths out my crumpled emotions.

My mother calls, "Dinner is ready!"

I put on jeans and a sweater. I pull down the sweater over my hip bone trying to poke a hole through the denim. A glance in the mirror shows darkening stubbles at the surgery site.

I'm not hungry, but she prepared my favorite dish—spaghetti with meatballs—and bought cookie dough ice cream. We eat so we don't have to talk. She discreetly watches me as I mechanically sprinkle parmesan cheese on my plate. Her face is stern—a sign she's about to say something important.

With her eyes down, she mutters, "You need to take better care of yourself. You can't just give up."

"Is that why you're here?" I yell back.

"Control your temper, Annie."

"I'm not like you, Mom! I'm not made of steel and stone!"

"I'm not made of steel and—" She chokes on her words.

I'm taken aback. It's the first time I see my mother cry.

"Do you know why we didn't adopt other children? We didn 't think we could love any child as much we loved you," she says through tears. "The thought of losing you is not something I can live with."

She gets up and walks to the box of tissues; when she returns, all sobered up, tears wiped off, she 's my mother again.

"You can 't stay locked up in here forever," she decrees, standing in front of me. Her tone is now more professorial and commanding. "You need your medication adjusted, you need vision therapy to strengthen the muscles in your left eye. You of all people know that you need counseling. I'll make some calls tomorrow."

My mother's healing plan is a code for "I love you and I won't let cancer take you away from me." She always approached motherhood with the same resolve she put into her career. My mother—CEO of Mothers, Inc.

Unable to fall asleep, I spend the night weighing the solutions available to me, but none of them will make a significant difference. They're palliative tools to escort patients to a peaceful end. I already vetoed conventional treatment. That leaves holistic therapies with anecdotal success rates and without clinical trials. No guarantee of success but without side effects.

After the last appointment with another oncologist, who confirmed I was doomed without radiation and chemo, we get back in the car. My mother's face changes color. She puts the key in the ignition but doesn't crank the engine. Her jade green eyes turn aquamarine as she stares in the distance through the rays of sunlight bouncing off the windshield.

"You can't accept this. There's gotta be a way we can fight it."

When my mother wants something, God himself has to obey. She never hears the word no. "You can't" means it's possible; "impossible" means try harder.

"My head is rotting, Mom. In a few months, I'll be drooling and babbling."

"Feeling sorry for yourself is pathetic. People beat the odds all the time. Why can't you be one of them?"

To anyone else, her words may sound harsh, but I know it's a hug. Those are her "I love you" words. A laugh bursts free. "I love you, Mom."

She glares and starts the car. "Where would you like to go for lunch?"

Translation: "I love you, too."

Before leaving me alone once more, she makes me a list of holistic centers to call. Her determination and my limp hope combine to an average effort.

My first call is to my colleague and friend Janet to ask for counseling. I've known Janet since grad school. She 's a brilliant psychologist, but she has given up her practice and mostly writes for psychology journals while she 's raising her two boys.

She's the first person I discuss cancer with, after Daniel and my parents. Words don 't flow easily. Telling others I'm defective is admitting to failure.

"What is going on exactly? You're the most stable person I know. Doctor Annie Seylor doesn't need counseling. She giggles. "Are you in love with the wrong guy?"

After a long pause, I manage to murmur, "I have cancer."

It's her turn to be on mute. People's reaction to cancer is unlike any other disease. It makes them uncomfortable. But as a professional, Janet comes back with the right response: "How are you feeling?"

"I need assistance to accept it happened to me and move through the grief phases. At the moment, all I feel is anger and depression."

Janet knows the last thing I want to talk about is cancer. So, in our weekly online sessions, we mostly talk about our memories of grad school. We reminisce about evenings spent at the library, our special Fridays, which consisted of pepperoni pizza and cheap beer, and our dates or the lack of them—like when we celebrated Valentine's together and the waiter thought we were lesbians. She talks about her children and her dog, and I share my memories of Fred. Mentioning Daniel is too painful. Janet takes me back to the past and then escorts me to a new present. Even though the future is a mystery, she helps me find the necessary ataraxia to live in the moment.

"Everyone makes plans about the future. Sometimes, the future is years away; sometimes, it's only a few months. But nobody knows how much time they have."

"Except, I do know."

"Not necessarily. Your tumor may regrow right away, or it may take years. But if you have only a few months, do you want to waste them?"

I keep the house as clean as my mother left it. I avoid mirrors and keep the bathroom light dim. I alternate between feeling peaceful and sad. Every morning, I study the calendar and count the number of days since my last conversation with Daniel. I wait for time to soothe the pain of losing him—it's in no hurry.

As we move through therapy, the rage slowly recedes and makes space for despondency. I tally the events of the recent months. The small window I had into happiness is now closed forever. The better I feel mentally, the more I miss him. It also dawns on me that I may never have another shot at love. The temptation to call him creeps up once in a while, but fear shackles me. My hollow eyes, partly shaved head, and gaunt face remind me to let go.

Eight weeks post-surgery seems like a year. On the surface, I'm getting stronger. Internally, the decay is probably forging ahead. My hair has grown enough to cover the scar, but not enough to go out without cover. I sit by the windowsill, sipping my morning tea while watching the squirrel steal the bird seeds I put in the flower pot. I contemplate calling the holistic centers my mother has selected. The phone interrupts my train of thought. Calls at 8:00 a.m. are unusual; a glance on the screen displays "Unknown." Someone in India is worried about my car warranty. I answer at the second ring.

"Buenos días," says the cheerful familiar voice. My heart drops. I can't breathe.

"Annie? Are you there?"

"Yes... Yes, I'm here."

"How are you?"

"You called my father."

It's all I can come up with after not talking to him for over a month. He feels so far away in time, like those faded photographs from the last century. Thankfully, he makes a joke of it.

"And I'll do it again if you don't behave."

"I don 't know what to say. I was..."

"Cara, you don 't have to apologize. I was prepared. I knew what was happening."

"Why do you love me so much?"

"This is only the beginning."

I sob uncontrollably. Unable to comfort me physically, he waits for me to catch my breath. Embarrassed, I rush to explain. "It 's the medication. It makes me feel weak and weepy."

"Hmm, that means I can take advantage of you. I'm getting on the next plane."

His sense of humor puts an end to the tears but opens a floodgate to guilt and remorse.

^ ^ ^

I'm not ready. My hair still has not grown enough to get an even haircut; I'm not motivated to mask the pallor with makeup; bursts of energy get quickly drowned in fatigue. But he insists on a video date.

I put on a mask and haul myself to the mall to buy the sexiest hat I can find. An elegant red wide-brim wool and felt hat that drops mid-ear and slightly above the eyebrows. A short black lace veil hangs just below the eyes. I put on some blush, red lipstick, and a pearl choker my parents gave me for my twentieth birthday. As I clasp the necklace around my neck, I'm thrown back to that day. It was more than a birthday. It was a celebration of a future full of promise.

I'd just graduated from college summa cum laude; I had been accepted to Harvard to pursue a doctorate in psychology to study trauma and recovery. Some nights, I was so excited about all the things I wanted to accomplish, I waited for the day to rise. Tuned to my emotions, Fred stayed up as well. I went to the kitchen to give him treats. I can still feel his joy as he followed me down the stairs.

I put on earrings and consult the mirror one last time before sitting at the computer. He joins the video from his office. He has a joyful disposition and looks irresistible in a designer navy blue suit with a light purple tie peppered with red and yellow motifs. It's the beginning of summer in Argentina, so his skin is a little darker, with deeper gold tones. Behind him is a large abstract painting by Emilio Pettoruti. Below the painting, on a credenza, stands a small glass sphere with a stainless steel bottom and long legs. It resembles a space capsule, but it's an airport terminal he designed years ago for some Middle Eastern country. Every time I peek inside his life, I fall in love a little deeper. At times, I feel a pinch in the gut. He's so accomplished and I'm just a psychologist with a couple of discounted books nobody reads.

"You look stunning! The curse of Tantalus. That's cruel, you know!"

"Glad you like my Princess Diana look."

"You don't need a hat. I love *you*, not just your hair."

"I think you love my legs."

"Precisely. Hair is easy, but you can't buy a nice pair of legs. Especially a pair like yours."

"What are your plans for Christmas?" I ask.

"We're having family over. My parents, my sister and her family. We'll keep it low key. Tanya wants to prepare the meal. I convinced her to just make dessert. How about you?"

"I'm staying home. But I'll be decorating. This house is going to look more festive than the mall."

He pauses, puts his chin on the back of his hand, and adopts a more serious tone. "You know, if travel was open, I'd be spending Christmas with you."

"Really? How about your family?"

"There is no way I'd let you spend Christmas alone in isolation. But no one can get out of Argentina at the moment."

"There will be other times. Once Argentina allows travel again, maybe we can schedule another scuba trip. I've been salivating over pictures of the Maldives on Instagram."

"We should plan a trip to Dubai. COVID is well controlled

there. They have huge aquariums for scuba diving. We could also attend a camel race."

"Aren't camels slow-moving animals?"

"They can be trained to run. The camel jockeys are as small as horse jockeys."

I listen to his stories of Dubai, the desert, and free-running gazelles and his voice wraps and soothes me like a lullaby.

Before we end our session, he silently studies my face for a second, as if he wants to take a mental picture. The blush on my cheeks gives my skin a reassuring glow and the elegant hat projects an image of health and glamor.

^^^

The internet abounds with healing centers, raw food, yoga, and fasting retreats. Scattered all over the world are institutes that specialize in cancer, from Australia to Israel, Mexico, and Japan. My mother selected the ones close to home so she and my Dad could visit: Florida, California, and Mexico. The one in Mexico is the only one that has a record of treating cancer patients. Their treatment method consists of megadoses of vitamin C injections and laetrile—no mention of nutrition or fasting.

We're nine months into the pandemic, if we count since the lockdown in March, and there is no end in sight. Dr. Fauci recommends we stay home, but airports will still be crowded. So, any travel plans will have to wait until after Christmas—the first one I'll spend alone. My mother insists we dine together virtually. We'll cook a Virginia ham, mashed potatoes, roasted beets, and she'll bake an apple pie, while mine will be baked by Marie Callender. A Zoom session with Daniel is planned for the evening.

Another area of study for psychologists and sociologists will emerge from this era. I open my laptop to jot down a few notes on possible topics of research: *Impact of isolation on school children; pandemic-related PTSD; escalation of domestic abuse; Healthcare workers and PTSD.*

∧∧∧

Santa Claus drives a UPS truck and he's been dropping off gifts since mid-December. I only have a two-foot-tall Christmas tree on the buffet with miniature ornaments hanging from its twigs, so I put the gifts in a corner of the living room next to the window, ready to be opened on Christmas Day. I received three packages from my parents, two from Daniel, one from Uncle Bob and Aunt Lydia, and one from Aunt Bettie.

Christmas Day, I wake up with the same anticipation I did as a child. My parents always greeted me like a star when I came downstairs. Watching me open gifts, they were as excited as I.

Christmas was my mother's favorite holiday. The tree was always stacked with gifts, and every inch of the house was decorated: wreaths on doors and dining room table, Santa dolls on furniture, potpourri, candles. I still smell the cinnamon aroma that filled every room. Other family members would arrive late in the morning, and we'd open gifts again. For breakfast, my mother served risengrynsgrøt, a Norwegian pudding offered with cinnamon. It's cooked with one almond and whoever found it in their bowl won a prize. My cousins and I would immediately furrow through our helpings in search of the almond. When we were little, my mother put three almonds in the pudding, violating her ancestral tradition.

WhatsApp beeps. Daniel sends his picture with a large smile, pointing at his sweatshirt with a message: *Feliz Navidad Amor y Salud.* I respond with hearts and kisses. He's surrounded by a lot of people and cannot escape for a chat. Like a teenager, he had to hide to text me. His Christmas is probably a big celebration in the Catholic tradition. I imagine a large family reunion, a long table with fancy china, crystal stemware, and flowers, a dominating Christmas tree engulfed with packages of all sizes wrapped in gold and silver gift paper. A twinge in my gut catches me by surprise; he's fully anchored in my life. I'm a footnote in his. But without him, I wouldn't experience this kind of love. A constant cognitive dissonance in our relationship.

I'll have to wait until evening for our video date and our gift opening time. I sent him a package with gourmet Virginia peanuts, vegan beef jerky—which he loves but cannot find in Argentina—and a Washington Capitals hat. Baseball hats are all the rage in Argentina.

I cook my Christmas dinner to enjoy virtually with my parents. I simmer a pot of cider with the usual spices and pineapple juice to replicate my grandmother's recipe, but it never tastes as good as hers. Nonetheless, the house smells like Christmas and, if I close my eyes, I can see all of it, the way it was before the pandemic, before cancer. A bygone era when people celebrated holidays, enjoyed weddings, and gathered at funerals.

A little after 2:00 p.m., we meet on Zoom. The same faces that populate my memory are now nested into little squares on a computer screen. They're sitting around their respective Christmas trees, so we can all open our gifts together. Despite the remoteness of the event, it still feels festive. The spirit of Christmas has gone digital.

After we all open our gifts, we lift our glasses to curse 2020. We wish for its joyful exit and to never return.

My parents and I remain on the Zoom call to share the holiday dinner, my mother complaining I did not use a more festive tablecloth.

"Annie, these rituals help people move through time and reconnect." That's her code for "I miss you." She gets misty-eyed and looks up to roll back the tears.

"I'm the psychologist. Leave the interpretation of human behavior to me." I move the computer to the buffet to show my miniature Christmas tree. "See, I have a tree."

"Are those gifts or earrings?" my father jokes, mocking the minuscule boxes hanging from the tiny branches.

"My tree is a girl and she's festive."

"Is your tree Brazilian? The only language where trees are feminine."

"I think she grew up in West Virginia."

Halfway through the meal, I disable the video and move to the couch to lie down. I listen to them and talk with my eyes closed. I eventually mumble "Merry Christmas" and drift into a heavy sleep.

Like a summer breeze, the nap gives me a small burst of energy, just enough to prepare for another Zoom show. I put on a white sweater with small green and red Christmas trees and a Santa hat for good measure. I apply makeup to mask the gray, tired skin tone before opening the video.

To speed up the clock, I go back to the mirror to check my appearance, reapply lipstick, and adjust my hair. It's our first Christmas *together* and I want it to be a happy memory. One where I'm healthy and radiant. Despite the geographical distance, his presence in my life fills the emptiness created by COVID and sweetens the bitterness of cancer. I ignore all the reasons we're not sharing the same space and reassure myself it's temporary.

This is perhaps the biggest difference between humans and animals. We're the only creatures who lie to ourselves and believe our own lies. So, to hold on to happiness and stay in the Christmas mood, I blame COVID for our physical separation.

We both enter the virtual room fifteen minutes early. He takes a good look at me and laughs at my silly hat.

"How was your Christmas? How many guests did you have?"

"The usual. Tanya baked her first pastafrola." He immediately moves his attention to the box of gifts I sent him.

When my turn comes to open the gifts, he asks that I open the little box last. I place the large rectangular box on my lap and tear through the wrapping. I first open the card, which has a poem in Spanish, so I ask for a translation.

"For a look, I would give a world; for a smile, I would give heaven…" He slows down the pace and recites the last line with a fervent tone. He looks me in the eyes through the camera and delivers the punchline: "But what would I give for chocolate?"

I burst into a loud laugh. "I was thinking what a horrible poem!"

"What can I say, I'm an architect, not a poet."

I want to say "I love you," but the words won't come out.

The box contains two layers of different shapes of chocolates: flat rectangles, white squares, and domes sprinkled with tiny pieces of nuts. I taste the square, which melts into a sweet cream as soon as it lands on my tongue.

"Delicious."

"And a hundred percent vegan. They're made in Bariloche. It's a town in Patagonia, considered the South American capital of chocolate."

I bring the little box to my ear and shake it, weigh it in my hand, and study its contours, before guessing its content—probably jewelry. When I finally open it, I retrieve a delicate velveteen pouch that feels a little heavy. I pull out a green necklace made of small sprigs of oval leaves and minuscule buds between them. Each leaf has a tiny bud at its base that's terminated by a freshwater pearl. I put it on and the delicate leaves rest on my collarbones. I run to the mirror, take off the Christmas hat, shake my head to realign my hair, and come back to face the camera.

"It goes perfectly with my red hair and would accentuate any décolleté."

"When I saw it, it reminded me of you. Strong, yet delicate."

We open our bottles of bubbly beverages and toast Christmas.

ΛΛΛ

The week between Christmas and the first day of the year is undoubtedly the most boring time. Gift-wrapping paper lingers on the floor next to open boxes. My inbox stopped chirping—even spammers are on a holiday break. The suitcase I opened yesterday lies empty in the living room. Two cups of tea are not enough to pull me out of indolence—until the phone vibrates.

"Good morning, Mom."

"Are you packed?"

"I started."

"Are you sure it's okay for you to travel so far?"

"I'm medically cleared to travel."

"I don't see why you have to go all the way to Argentina when there are so many places around here."

"Daniel said it's one of the best centers for holistic cancer treatment and it's secluded."

"I don't like the sound of this."

"It's only for three months."

"All right. Don't forget to take good quality masks and a hand sanitizer. I'll send you anything you need. Have a safe trip and let us know when you get there."

ΛΛΛ

January is the peak of summer in the Southern Hemisphere. The plane glides through a sunny blue sky approaching Ezeiza International Airport around lunchtime.

Shortly before landing, I head to the bathroom to change clothes and adjust my makeup. A concealer under the eyes hides the purple; blush and lipstick for a fresher look. I want to stretch those last few minutes so time can help improve my appearance and appease the anxiety, but a flight attendant knocks on the door and orders me back to my seat.

I'm still uncertain if I made the right decision coming to Argentina, but he vetoed my first choice— the healing center in Mexico—and insisted I go to Años Mejores in the Province of Jujuy instead. The infection rate there is low due to heat, open spaces, and people's willingness to obey COVID rules. He has a connection who will lobby for us to allow him to visit.

Años Mejores has been treating cancer patients for twenty years. Aside from nutrition therapy, the program includes meditation, yoga, and a Japanese self-healing technique called *Jin Shin Jyutsu*. So, I brace myself for three months of vegan meals with sprouts, celery juice, and different warrior positions.

Carry-on bag slung over my shoulder, purse in the crook of my arm, I wheel the suitcase to the exit. My mouth is dry, my mid-section fluffy and porous like a sponge. I struggle to walk straight on wobbly legs. All the suffering of the last few months has lumped inside my chest, causing my alveoli to constrict.

He's the first face I see in the small crowd. His beaming smile, visible behind the mask, instantly erases the time we were apart. Only this moment exists, and I can breathe again. He takes my carry-on to lift it onto his shoulder and squeezes me firmly against his chest. I give in to the strength of his grasp and let my head rest on his shoulder, swayed by his voice as he breathes through the mask and into my hair. "Bienvenida a Argentina, mi amor!"

On the way to the hotel, he drives with one hand while holding mine with the other. The highway is lined with apartment and office buildings, small towns, and shopping centers.

"After you get some rest, I'll give you a tour of the city. Just so you know, food is not great in Buenos Aires."

"You mean, no burgers?"

"Oh, there are plenty of burgers. But restaurants are rather mediocre."

"We'll live on love and wine then."

"Wine is excellent here. As for love, I got you covered."

/\ /\ /\

The Hyatt in Recoleta looks like a palace, hence the name, Palacio Duhau. The front facade overlooks a palm tree and rows of white roses and red peonies. The taxi driver opens the door for us to exit while a man in uniform with a cart rushes to take our luggage. Two doormen greet us and show us to the lobby.

"Are you some kind of celebrity?"

"How d'you mean?"

"The way everyone reacts around us."

He squeezes my hand, turns toward me, and holds his gaze on my face for a second. Uncomfortable, I look away. I'm like that rotten fruit: ripe and shiny on the outside while a worm is devouring it inside.

"They're reacting to you. They think you're a Hollywood star."

After we register, we take the elevator to our room, where our luggage has already been delivered. The room is spacious, with large windows that generously pour in sunlight. White sheers cover the glass while red velvet curtains are drawn to the sides. A divan stuffed with pillows rests against the wall facing the bed, brightened by a side table with a vase of fresh tropical flowers. I remove my shoes and give in to the lure of the inviting king-size bed tucked against the wall next to the marble bathroom.

"Do you want lunch? We can go out or order room service." He awkwardly stands next to the door, looking at the carpet.

"No, I just want to rest for a minute. Come sit next to me."

He lies down facing me, his fingers searching through my hair and finding the outline of the scar hidden there. He lowers his voice, as if he doesn't want to be heard, and asks if it hurts. He softly kisses my forehead, then my left cheek; he slowly moves down to my lips. He nibbles, waiting to be invited. Feeling no resistance, he gradually covers my entire mouth with a molten kiss that intensifies my craving for more.

I hold him tight to convince myself that this is all real and to reassure him everything will be all right. It's the kind of hug that denies the fragility of life. I press my chest against his to get even closer. His warmth, his gentle touch, and his love ignite me. Chemical signals travel through my nerves like lightning. The sparks accelerate my pulse and empower my grip. I grab his face and voraciously invade his mouth, pressing his face against mine. Then, I run my hands over his chest, under the shirt; I get a hold of the buttons and start to pull on them to undress him. He gently pulls away and cups my frenzied hands inside his. Feeling caught, I recoil.

"Are you sure this is okay?" he asks.

I bury my face in his chest. "It's my head that's rotten. The body's fine."

"You shouldn't talk like that."

"I need to get all the sarcasm out of my system before I have to sing OM every day."

He kisses me to silence my negativity.

What he doesn't know is I *can* have sex, I just don't know if I'll enjoy it. But it's the kind of information I keep to myself. So far, I can feel and my libido is intact. For the rest, many women say it's optional—only because they don't know any better.

His left hand cradles my head while his right massages the crown. His body presses down on mine as he kisses me deeper. He then moves down my neck, my breasts, and explores every inch of my body, kissing and touching, leaving no part unloved. Like a creek after the rain, I'm whole and singing again.

I snuggle against him. "Houston, we don't have a problem."

He nibbles on my shoulder. "Dr. Lorenzo's post-surgery therapy."

"Five-star review."

We get dressed and with masked faces, we leave the room. We stroll down to the terrace for a late lunch. The pandemic and the hour of the day provide for many available tables. As soon as we sit down, a waiter brings us menus, deploys the white umbrella, and disappears.

Our table overlooks a canopy of grass that resembles a Persian rug. A wave of happiness sweeps over me like a fog engulfing a mountain in the spring. I get swayed into a lullaby by the delicate perfume of the flowers and the chirping of birds, blending into the rainbow of colors to complete the vacation atmosphere. He holds my hand on the table and looks at me in silence.

"I'm not complaining, but your demeanor is different. Is that due to the surgery?"

"That, my darling, is another symptom of brain surgery: sexual aggression."

"I need to call Años Mejores and have them evacuate the men!"

"Cancer! Turns out, it's hysterical." A rush of blood heats my cheeks, probably turning them as red as the peonies. As an apology, I offer an explanation.

"Sometimes, it's the reverse. The patient has no libido or feels nothing during intercourse. It's worse for men because they can't pretend."

"Are there any treatments?"

"Not really. People often develop a heightened sexual appetite or depression due to loss of desire or impotence. But sexual activity is still taboo, so they never complain."

"This is common and nothing can be done about it?"

"Doctors only treat tumor growth. Quality of life is irrelevant to them. We're left to fend for ourselves in the wilderness that's life after cancer."

"Is this why you refused the treatment?"

"Not exactly. Radiation therapy kills both cancerous and healthy cells. I'd have severe memory loss, possibly speech impairment, and chemo always alters biochemistry. The symptoms could take years to develop."

"Aren't those changes temporary?"

"It depends on how much damage is done and how the body recovers. Everybody's different. No way to predict."

The waiter brings our drinks and takes our order. The

steak is tempting, but I opt for a quinoa salad with grilled green papaya. He orders a roasted pineapple with chimichurri sauce, a green salad, and patatas bravas to share.

Patatas bravas are perhaps the best Spanish invention. The potatoes are cut into small chunks and fried. They're crunchy on the outside, creamy inside, and served with a dipping sauce made of roasted tomatoes and spices. The flavor of the sauce and the sweetness of the potatoes are a perfect marriage that makes the palate sing. I pile them in my mouth one by one to the last bite. He probably ate two or three pieces. He looks at me with a fatherly attitude.

"I guess I was hungrier than I thought."

"Glad you got your appetite back. You need to gain some weight."

After the meal, I'm overcome by fatigue. Instead of exploring Buenos Aires, we return to the room. He cautions me not to fall asleep and to hang on until evening. He pulls out his laptop to show me the itinerary he has planned for us to travel to Años Mejores.

"It's a two-hour flight to Jujuy. Then, we'll rent a car. We'll stop in San Salvador de Jujuy for lunch. I found a nice restaurant that's open. After lunch, you can decide which of these locations you want to visit." He shows me two brochures: Termas de Reyes or Laguna de Yala.

Termas de Reyes, a majestic landscape with hills and valleys, inspire awe and reverence for nature. I flip through glossy pictures of the long mountain range separated by the Reyes River, reminiscent of the Hawai'ian islands with round back hills covered with luscious green grass. Alternating anticline and syncline folds with limbs plunging into the river. Too tired to hold the brochure, I close my eyes on the hot springs and steaming pools. I fall asleep, sinking into the beauty of Argentina.

/\ /\ /\

After collecting our luggage and rental car, we leave the

airport and head for San Salvador. La Ruta 40 cuts through farmland along the Rio Grande River to Palpala, a quaint little village with colonial architecture and a small church tucked at the foothills of a multicolor mountain flowing with curtains of rocks from a blue sky, topped with a couple of fluffy white clouds.

We take a driving break.

"The clouds over the mountains look like vanilla ice cream."

"Does this mean you're hungry?" he replies, pulling me closer.

"I'm in a sweet mood."

"Argentina agrees with you."

I photograph the front facade of the church with its arcades, arched windows, and a dome-shaped bell tower mounted with a cross that reaches high in the sky. We meander around the court, then enter through the tall paneled doors into the nave. He kneels to make the sign of the cross.

We amble to the altar with our hands interlaced. Stained-glass quatrefoil windows shine on us with their gold, ruby, and sapphire hues. We stop at the round votive candle stand stacked with garnet-red cups where small candles sacrifice their wax. To the right of the altar, a life-size statue of the Virgin Mary looks down at vases of flowers. Daniel reaches into his pocket for coins that he then inserts into the slot of the candle stand in exchange for a candle to light. We stare in silence at the little flames and inhale the aroma of burning wax blended with the scent of old wood.

I can count on my fingers the times I've been in a church: playing tourist in a couple of European cathedrals, a couple of weddings, and one funeral. Every time I look at Jesus with his hands and feet nailed to the cross, I wonder what kind of God would let his son undergo so much suffering and why such a God would be loving toward his followers.

"You know... I'm not sure I believe in God," I tell him as

we walk to the car.

"I'll believe for both of us and, when we go to mass, I'll get two Ostia."

"Do I have to go mass?"q

"Religion is not a requirement in Argentina, but soccer--"

"Do I have to hate Brazil, too?"

"It wouldn't hurt."

I laugh with the innocence of a tickled child before we lose ourselves in another communion kiss.

We arrive in San Salvador around lunchtime. We drive by the Plaza Belgrano, the location of the government house—a beautiful large building in the typical colonial style architecture, engulfed in blooming leafy shrubbery and palm trees with a large fountain basin in the front shooting geysers. We cut through Bario Centro to reach Independencia and arrive at Viracocha, the restaurant he selected.

The outside of the restaurant looks like a shack—a plain building with a pale pink facade without decorations or anything to suggest it houses a dining establishment. An old piece of broken wood with the name Viracocha hangs from heavy rusted chains above the door.

Once inside, it's like stepping somewhere into old Europe. A cavernous interior similar to those underground restaurants in Eastern Europe is filled with rustic furniture; shelves exhibit terracotta objects; a long hallway divided by red brick archways separates dining rooms; tables are draped with white tablecloths topped with runners in the Quechua design pattern. It's a utopian atmosphere where romance meets magic. The waiter leads us through the archways to our table in the back—Daniel always insists on corner tables, away from spectators.

The romantic atmosphere, his presence, and the exotic decor create a fairy tale picture tainted with despair. Cancer is an invisible witch with infinite powers. I would like for time to stop here—life may never be this beautiful again.

The waiter brings us menus and speaks in Spanish.

"Dos aguas sin gas por favor," Daniel replies.

We spend two hours on lunch. Argentinian waiters have their own timetable. It's hard to discern whether the food is delicious or if I'm just grateful to be served.

After lunch, I feel life draining out of me. My entire body is a heavy shapeless mass crushed under a blanket of hot lava that melts my bones. I'm afraid I'll stumble if I stand. "Honey, I don't think I'll enjoy the hot springs."

"It's only thirty minutes away. There is a nice hotel there. We could get a room to take a nap?"

"No, I'll sleep in the car. Let's just drive to the center. It would be nice to arrive during daylight."

It's not the kind of fatigue that can be cured by a nap. Lying down provides relief but doesn't lead to restorative sleep. I drag myself to the car and collapse onto the seat.

As we drive up Route 9, he turns into a tourist guide. The culture in Jujuy is autochthonous. Unlike the rest of Argentina, which emulates Europe more than South America, Jujuy still holds many pagan rituals as dominant. It's a mostly Andean culture where force-feeding animals, offerings to the Gods, and coca leaf blessings are common practice. People rely more on shamans and botanical remedies than modern medicine.

"How come they have so many churches?"

"They didn't have a say in the matter. A lot of these churches were built during the colonial era."

I listen to his voice like a lullaby and blink incessantly to keep my eyes open.

"Are you feeling dizzy?"

"No, just tired."

"I'll stop talking so you can rest."

I open my eyes when he turns left onto Route 52 toward Purmamarca. The road winds through switchbacks over a rough and dry terrain. I sit up to avoid motion sickness and look out of the window to see a Martian terrain. Everything below the sky is salmon-colored, with touches of brown and purple ribbons in the distance. It's the majestic Quebrada de

Humahuaca with its multicolored hills. I check the gas tank. It's half full. The striking beauty of the wilderness is a delight to the eye but a menace to human life dependent on water and shelter from the sun.

"Is this where you're going to murder me?"

"That's the plan," he says, without taking his eyes off the road.

"I'll come back to haunt you. I'll terrorize all your dates."

He's amused by the idea of "dates." He gives me his usual half smile while extending his arm to put his fingers through my hair.

We arrive at the pre-Hispanic Quechuan village of Purmamarca mid-afternoon. Cradled in these rocky mountains for over four centuries, its roads have not undergone modern construction. I try to identify all the colors of the round-back hills, layered like a carefully crafted art piece.

Since we arrived earlier than expected, he takes a small detour into Plaza 9 de Julio to show me an iconic tree. We turn onto a street called Florida, which drops us on the outskirts of the Plaza.

We walk into the famous square, right into the market, amid stacks of wool blankets, ponchos, sweaters, scarves, and various articles of clothing bursting with rainbow colors and neatly lined up, baking in the sun. Masked Quechua women with their little round hats and sweat-moist faces sit on the ground chatting while waiting for customers. In the background, small souvenir shops overflow with objects from tiny wooden carved cacti, statues, and guitars, to kitchen utensils.

We come to the famous Algarrobo tree. It's more than the eye can capture: a giant octopus with tentacles reaching left, right, and upward, all waving their little bundles of wispy leaves in the sky. The enormous trunk is about thirty feet in diameter. The naked branches and the trunk have the texture of dried cat's claw twigs—brownish-red, fibrous, and flaky. One branch twisting around the trunk forms an eye. The others twist and turn and hug each other or fuse into one large arm. I take pictures from all angles to capture its majesty, but I can't fit the whole tree into one frame.

"This tree is seven hundred years old," Daniel says.

"It's older than Argentina."

"Legend has it, the famous General Belgrano rested under its shade."

I perk up as we approach Años Mejores. It has the allure of a small hotel, with only twenty rooms at the foothills of the multicolored hills. Its conspicuous architecture blends harmoniously with its surrounding landscape and culture. Pink and purplish small cabins are built with local materials—cactus wood, stone, and clay. A winding stony path that cuts through a square surrounded by individual rooms takes us to the reception desk. Each corner of the square is guarded by a tall fat cactus while smaller versions accessorize the front door of each guest room.

From the outside, the reception office looks exactly like all the other rooms, but with a *Recepción* sign above the door. A short young woman with glasses and greasy hair hanging on her shoulders greets us with a "Bienvenidos a Años Mejores."

She takes our temperatures and addresses Daniel in Spanish before switching to English. She sizes me up and gives me her warmest smile. "Ooh, Estadounidense! I go to America tree jears before, to Florida."

She presents me with the bylaws of the center and a stack of forms to fill out. Some rules are standard—no smoking, no alcohol, no drugs; others are most unusual—no perfume and no outside food. The prohibition of perfume is because it bothers the fasters. As for the food, it's to ensure that all residents stick to a clean vegan diet without toxic ingredients. We're to stay in the compound and never venture out unless accompanied. No visitors are allowed unless pre-approved by management. Another sheet of paper includes a map of the compound and its different facilities: dining room, yoga studio, massage station, and recreation room with television.

Dizzy and weak, I skim the rest of the documents. I sign and give the papers back to Miss Florida. She hands me a key and a schedule for the next day. She goes over meal times and other activities, then instructs me to be in my room at 10:00 a.m. the next day. A member of the staff will come to escort me to the orientation. She tells Daniel he has to say goodbye here. He isn't allowed in the compound beyond the reception desk, even with a mask.

He brings my luggage in, and I walk him back to the car. A chill runs over my body. The surrounding beauty of the landscape takes on an oppressive hospital feel—a voluntary incarceration. It's a brutal transition from life as a couple to being left behind. We savor a few last minutes inside the car.

"You're going to leave me here alone."

"I'm going to drive back alone."

I forgot that a long road awaits him. Being in a foreign environment reduces people to selfish children. We hug for a long time. I refuse to let go. He withdraws and holds my face in his hands. "You'll like it here. They're very genuine people."

"And *vegan*!"

5 - The Hill of Seven Colors

The sun streams through the small round window. In the absence of blinds or curtains to shield the room from the perky morning brightness, the sun serves as an alarm clock. I stagger into the shower—a corner with a large bowl to stand in, surrounded by a thin plastic curtain. The water is cold. I let it run and step out.

Waiting for the water to heat, I pull out the map of the complex from the stack of paperwork and locate the dining area. Exhausted from the trip, my tired body had succumbed to sleep immediately the previous night, leaving me no time to become oriented with my surroundings.

I return to the shower, now steaming hot, and float in the aroma of the mango shower gel my mother gave me. I linger a little before shutting off the water and stepping out. I towel off, slip into my floral maxi dress with front buttons, and head to the dining area.

The outdoor dining space is a pavilion with a gable roof and white curtains hanging from each corner beam. I follow the alley to the right of the dining room, bordered by cacti and blooming plants. Beyond the alley, the outdoor kitchen forms an L shape with the dining room. Several masked individuals lay out trays of food, bowls of fruit, jugs of water, bottles of juice, and hot coffee, while a group of people chats away on the other side of the pool.

I approach the kitchen counter to introduce myself and a tall woman with shiny black hair greets me. She's wearing a white apron with "Chef Laora" embroidered under the Años Mejores logo. She gestures to her face and repeats "mascarilla, mascarilla" and hands me a mask.

"I'm sorry, I forgot."

She switches to English. "Annie?" She grins. "You arrived last night. I don't have your paperwork yet. Do you want coffee or tea?"

"Tea, please."

She hands me an empty cup and shows me a basket of teabags. *Passionflower-ginger. Here's something I never had before.* I drop the teabag in a cup and pour boiling water over it.

I proceed toward the small masked crowd waiting for breakfast. They're conversing and laughing; I move toward them with the steps of a chained prisoner. A newfound awareness shakes me: I'm one of them: a patient. My jaw clenches as the words "sick" and "cancer" clang in my head.

Everyone welcomes me with the same demeanor one would expect from old friends. At first glance, none of them looks sick. It's a resort atmosphere rather than a healing center for the damaged and defective. *Stay positive, Annie!*

Ernesto is the first to introduce himself. A tall Argentinian man with a good command of English and a strong accent. He's wearing a bathing suit and a towel around his neck, long enough to cover his protruding belly. His flirtatious attitude is unexpected and refreshing.

"Good morning, I'm Annie. I arrived late yesterday."

"Annie! Welcome. Are you a model?" he asks.

The woman next to him elbows him in the side. "Hello, Annie. I'm Donna. I'm the model. From California."

Donna is probably in her late fifties. Long blonde hair frames her puffy face and flows freely on her round shoulders. She's a beautiful woman with greenish-brown eyes and a small trumpet nose. She carries a few extra pounds around her belly, which she hides with a long purple shirt over white shorts.

Everyone laughs, except a small woman in the back. She holds a cup in one hand while the other twirls a long strand of hair. She looks at me with confused eyes. Ernesto turns to her and translates into Spanish, and her confusion clears.

"Where are you from, hon?" Donna asks with a warm smile.

"I live in Virginia."

"Beautiful state. I did my undergrad at UVA."

She puts her hand on my shoulder as she introduces me to the others. "This is Pablo. He's from Spain. Sylvia is from Italy, and Marta is from Germany. We are the United Patients!"

We do an elbow shake to comply with COVID rules. Before I start talking, Laora calls us to breakfast.

We gather in the dining area, around a heavy wooden table measuring about eight feet long with benches on each side and overlooking the swimming pool. An array of warm and cold mouth-watering dishes are arranged around an elegant flower bowl. Grain-free pancakes with organic birch syrup; harvest "omelet"—which Donna tells me tastes exactly like eggs; I salivate at the sight of bacon, but the ingredients card lists dried and seasoned jackfruit; the mushroom soup is all gray and not so appetizing. A mixed greens salad with papaya and mango has its own lime-avocado dressing. I put a small amount of each on my plate for sampling.

"The one thing we never complain about in this place is the food," says Donna as she fills her plate.

Ernesto chimes in. "That's why I keep coming back."

"I'll eat anything with bacon." I laugh back.

The omelet has an egg texture and flavor. The jackfruit is close but no cigar. It's chewy with a smoky flavor that hints at bacon, but not the same. The gluten-free rolls are soft and sweet. Mushroom soup for breakfast is a novelty, but it does pair well with the other dishes.

After breakfast, I return to my room—my home for the next three months—to wait for the 10:00 a.m. visit to learn about my treatment plan. I have to change my diet, learn about healing foods, listen to lectures, learn to cook, wait, and hope. After the wait, I will find out if my life has a definite expiration date. Then, there is the loss of income; if I have a future, what will it look like? How will COVID change the counseling landscape? A lot of my colleagues are conducting their sessions online. Will this become the norm?

My savings will last two years. But then again, I may not be here that long. Anxiety about the future does not brighten the present. I need to set everything aside and develop tools to cope with the confinement and ease the burden of the wait. Something I do very well—for other people.

My guide is at the door: a tiny woman in a white lab coat who looks not a day over fifteen. Wide-open brown eyes illuminate her face, adorned with modern plastic and metal glasses, so small and round they barely cover the eye, but give her an erudite aura. Her shiny black hair is tied in a bun, revealing beautiful small ears with diamond studs. She introduces herself as Karina Viridis, the nutritionist. She looks down at the stack of papers on her clipboard and back at me.

"You're Dr. Saylor? May I call you Annie? We use first names for everyone here."

She motions for me to follow. We walk through the reception office into a narrow dark hallway, then to a windowless office, not without a cactus. It's a dark room lit only by two lamps. She sits in an ergonomic chair behind a large desk facing two chairs. She gestures for me to sit. I spot a binder entitled "*patients*" on the credenza behind her. As she opens her laptop, I look at the canvas of photographs on the left wall. I am particularly drawn to a middle-aged man with a dignified forehead and a Robert DeNiro-type nose.

"That's Giovanni," she says with a glowing smile as she twists around to grab the binder. She opens it to different pictures of Giovanni. In one of them, he's sitting with his lower body covered with a blanket. "See, he's covering himself because his testicles are the size of a cantaloupe. He came here after he was diagnosed with prostate cancer." She effusively recounts how Giovanni came to the center after the medical establishment told him there was nothing they could do for him. They expected him to live less than a year, even if he underwent traditional treatment. Then she points at another picture where Giovanni is standing straight next to a tree, sunbathing. "This is him after three months on our program." She turns to another page. "And here, in his home in Italy, a year later. No swelling. Lab tests show PSA within normal range." She flips through the pages and shows me more pictures of patient success stories until I interrupt her.

"Have you treated anyone with a brain tumor?"

She lifts her eyes and smiles behind her mask. "You!" Then she continues with her lecture.

The thread of hope I was holding on to just shrank. She proceeds with her prepared questionnaire and asks about my lifestyle, any metabolic problems, digestive issues, and known allergies. Then she turns the page to the food section.

"What are your favorite foods and how often do you eat them?"

"Spaghetti with meatballs, steak, cheese. I eat meat about once a day to get enough protein."

Her sweet, cheerful face closes up. "Any fruit, vegetables, legumes?"

"I live alone and I don't know how to cook, so I rarely buy vegetables, but I eat them in restaurants."

Her expression darkens. "Animal foods create oxidative stress and increase the need for antioxidants."

She goes on and on about glycoxidation and lipoxidation end-products and the Maillard reaction. I keep my eyes on her serious face while what's left of my brain tunes her out. Then she hands me literature about the link between cancer and meat consumption.

"Clinical studies have found a positive association between meat consumption and brain tumors," she insists.

"So, I brought this on myself because I eat meat?"

"I'm just emphasizing that meat can be at the origin of carcinogenesis." She licks her dry lips and lowers her gaze to the desk. "This afternoon, you'll meet with Dr. Hidalgo. He'll give you more information about the program and what tests you need."

She hands me a binder with educational material and a card with a schedule of activities. She recommends I attend the cooking and nutrition classes. "I will put together a customized nutrition plan for you. The meals are the same for everyone, but we tweak the program slightly for each person depending on the health challenge."

She points at the activities schedule. "Here, you'll find all the program details and a listing of the daily activities. We added pictures of instructors since they are all masked. You're encouraged to wear a mask at all times as well, particularly when participating in group activities."

From the credenza behind her, she retrieves an assortment of supplements: vitamins, minerals, antioxidants, botanicals, and different nutrient combinations for each organelle inside human cells. She shows me a booklet about the supplements and how and when to take them.

"We will put the bag in your room. You can continue your tour hands-free." She opens the door and a tall, slender woman is already waiting.

"My name is Diana. Nice to meet you, Annie."

"Likewise."

Diana must be in her forties. She has short blonde hair and, on her badge picture, she smiles with fleshy lips over a row of perfect teeth. Her accent is enchanting.

"I'm the yoga teacher, but I also do the massages." Really, Diana seems to be a jack-of-all-trades. She's the meditation guru, massage therapist, and Jin Shin Jyutsu therapist. She even fills in when the receptionist needs a break.

"How long have you been working here?"

She laughs behind her mask, "As long as the owners. Fifteen years."

No doubt she has met every patient who ever passed through these doors and knows all the secrets and gossip.

"People come here tired and burdened by disease and stress. We cleanse their soul and fill them with hope. Everyone leaves a changed person," she says, swiping her hair to the back of her head.

She has her work cut out for her with me, as I'm currently hope-resistant.

As we walk through different parts of the compound, Diana gives me a detailed account of its history. It's the idea of a Japanese businessman whose daughter died from ovarian cancer. Chemotherapy made her sicker and failed to save her life. He hired a group of scientists to study nutrition as a tool to put cancer in remission. They developed a protocol involving fasting and a plant-based diet, and created a special antioxidant formula called *Kibō,* which means hope in Japanese. If antioxidants are not balanced properly, they could have adverse effects and encourage tumor growth instead of suppressing it.

"We've been using the same protocol for years. It ended up helping other patients with type 2 diabetes, autoimmune disease, and other dysfunctions that don't even have a name yet."

"How long does it take for this protocol to take effect?"

She replies to a text message before answering. "It varies from person to person. Dr. Hidalgo can probably tell you why. We've seen people reverse type 2 diabetes in as little as six weeks. We've had people with fibromyalgia who completely recovered in two weeks. A few people take longer, but the healing continues even after they leave."

"As long as they stay on the MicroRiche diet?"

"Exactly." Sensing my skepticism, she adds, "But that's not difficult. Once you experience good health, why would you go back?"

Outside, she shows me a narrow path bordered by willows. Not the willows we have back home, but short trees with blooms.

She extends her arm to point at the dirt path, "This is called Paseo de la Serenidad and is two kilometers long. Patients can walk all the way to the end. Beyond that is just brush leading to the hills."

We return inside the compound and enter the massage room. Lavender aroma wafts from the diffuser. The massage table in the center occupies most of the space. Coral and gold pillows line the walls in an alternating pattern. A tray of small, fragrant oil bottles on a velvet ottoman accent the room from the right corner. Diana recommends I get a massage at least once a week for relaxation and better sleep. We step out and she leads me to a bright room with large windows.

"This is the yoga studio." She presses down on the plunger of the disinfectant bottle by the door and smears the gel over her hands.

The yoga studio is a large room with pastel-painted walls decorated with Saraswati and lotus symbols. A stack of mats rests against the back wall and a tower of rolled towels is artfully positioned in the left corner.

"Yoga classes are twice a day: after breakfast, then candlelight yoga in the evening. Make sure you participate as often as you can. Yoga is the best way to detoxify the mind and usher in divine light."

I nod and silently chuckle at how everyone suffers from chemophobia in this place.

Facing the yoga studio is the recreation room. Large and cozy, it also serves as a library. Its walls are stacked with bookcases, tables hold magazines and games, and a large-screen television is mounted on the back wall. Diana points at couches and armchair and says, "We encourage all members to gather in this room for socializing and get to know each other. Building connections fosters healing and lightens your mood."

"As long as no one discusses politics." We laugh in agreement. Several drum stools in pastel colors dot the room and create a festive atmosphere. I sit on one to test it.

We leave the recreation room and walk outside to return to the dining area. It's lunchtime, an opportunity for a formal introduction to the kitchen staff. Sweet aromas of herbs and spices fill the air —an olfactory overload acting as an orexigenic.

Along with Chef Laora, AM has two maids who also help in the kitchen. "We all wear many hats here," Diana says. She introduces me to Stefani, who only speaks Spanish.

"Buenas tardes," Stefani says cheerfully.

Sonia is from Brazil and speaks decent Spanish and some English. "Welcum to Años Mejores."

They're both in their early twenties, beautiful with a

glow seen only in magazines. After the introductions, Diana takes me to the indoor dining room and shows me a refrigerator with water and different homemade juices, kombucha, and some non-dairy yogurt. On the table is another display of food: a basket of fruit and a tray of sugary treats—cocada, chocolate-walnut bars, and some seed and coconut balls. This section is open at all times for patients who need to snack any time of the day.

Diana reminds me to meet with Dr. Hidalgo at the same office where I met the nutritionist and wishes me luck. I thank her and head to the buffet. I can't say I'm hungry, but the artful display of food, makes my mouth water from both the visual and the olfactory stimulation.

Each food is served in its matching dish: glass bowls are used for salads to show off their colors, terracotta terrines to keep soups warm, and ornate ceramic dishes for optimal casserole baking and serving. A card is propped against each dish to list its ingredients.

The front of the buffet presents a row of soups and casseroles: Madrasa soup with lentils, goji berries, and mango powder; mushroom consommé; Rio Grande casserole made with black beans, quinoa, cilantro, topped with avocado and homemade crema. Riced cauliflower has been all the rage in the pas few years. Chef Laora prepared it with fermented vegetables and an Asian sauce. A less familiar food: macachin purée, tickles my curiosity. Salads are positioned behind the warm dishes. Mixed greens topped with strawberries, lychee, and pumpkin seeds; salad Niçoise tossed with olives and tomatoes and "chicken" salad made from jackfruit, salsify, and a creamy tahini dressing. I study the ingredients and try to imagine what they'll taste like together. I've never heard of jackfruit or salsify before, much less macachin.

Ernesto stands behind me and encourages me to take the first plate with an "Après vous!" His disarming smile lights his gold-brown eyes. His silver hair and his stooped silhouette show his age—probably seventy. It's his second visit to the center, though he jokes that he comes for the food. He was diagnosed with multiple myeloma three years ago. He cheerfully tells the story of how he announced it to his wife.

"I *tol kher* how would you like to have business, *khouse*, and find yourself younger man. She said 'you *khave* girlfriend."

Then he asks bluntly, "What is your type of cancer?"

I remove the scrunchy from my wrist and twist it around my hair to form a ponytail. "What type of business did you have?"

"I owned bakery. After cancer, I sold it and retired. I was very tired for too much months. Now, I spend time with grandchildren and travel with wife." He sighs and shakes a finger. "You know what I'm sad about?"

"Having cancer?"

He scratches his chin. "After cancer, doctor said limit activity and stress. So, I stop work. It open my eyes to all the years I put in work and never took vacation or weekend. So much life I missed. Thirty years. All given to bakery. I even worked on the eve of my son's wedding." His voice rises with pride. "I made a giant cake. It stood in chocolate lake and coconut cream as snowflakes." He opens his cell phone and scrolls through pictures of the cake.

His type of cancer was the most aggressive and only fifty percent of patients survived two to five years post-diagnosis. He endured the usual medical treatment, and as soon as it ended, he headed to AM. After three months, he returned home for more tests. The M protein was at a normal level. He was subsequently tested every six months with the same "joyful" results.

"I tried to give them brochure for other patients, but they brushed me off as stupid old man."

Sylvia arrives, fills her plate, and sits next to us. She's a beautiful woman in her late forties with curly black hair and almond-shaped brown eyes that say, *I'll tell the truth and nothing but the truth.* An English teacher in Milan, she speaks with a mixture of Italian and British accents which culminates into a melody. She introduces herself to me a second time and, before she asks what type of cancer I have, I beat her to the punch.

"So, what brought you here?"

"Liver cancer. I could not tolerate chemo, so my son combed the internet until he found this place. It's our last resort."

"You still have cancer then?"

"Not for long." She beams. "I've been here for one month. I'm no longer tired, no nausea after eating. Something is changing."

Postprandial fatigue creeps up turning my body into jello. I stand, excuse myself, and return to my room to rest before meeting with the famous doctor. Lying on the bed, I leaf through the paperwork to check the events list. Diana holds meditation sessions daily, Karina teaches cooking weekly, and Dr. Hidalgo lectures monthly. Massage and Jin Shin Jyutsu treatment are upon request and not included in the fee we already paid.

Every Monday at four, they serve what they call *"dessert and champagne."* Their version of champagne—kombucha with increased carbonation. Every Friday, they have a food theme where all the meals are inspired by a different country.

ΛΛΛ

Dr. Nick Hidalgo is a small, thin man in his early forties with soft oval eyes and a friendly face. A cascade of black locks forms a bonnet on his head. He greets me with a large smile, but no handshake—COVID oblige.

He looks at me with a frank and eager disposition. "I hear you're American. I went to UCLA and lived in California for ten years. Still have friends there."

"I thought I saw you in a few movies."

"You're funny. How do you like it here so far?"

"Can't complain. The staff is amazing, and the food

surpassed my expectations."

"We get that all the time. People think we live on seeds and sprouts." His warm and cuddly smile reminds me of Daniel.

He opens my medical history file and pulls out the nutritionist's report. A spasm takes over my face as I brace myself for another lecture about my diet.

"You have a very aggressive tumor. We're going to use several methods to attempt to stop its proliferation and hopefully kill it."

Dr. Hidalgo's words fall on me like the first drops of rain on a hot summer day, but I remain cautious in my enthusiasm. AM has not treated anyone with anaplastic astrocytoma.

"The surgeon couldn't remove all of it, so I'm told it'll regrow and fast. My life expectancy is less than a year."

"We'll change that," he says with calm confidence.

"So, why did this happen to me? Is it genetics, my diet, or just luck?"

"Genes are turned on and off when triggered by certain factors. Toxicity plays a major role, as do genetics, infections, and diet, being the biggest factor."

He pauses and flips through my files, then lifts up his beautiful brown eyes. "Most of the time, it's a combination of factors that cause disease. Diet is an important component because, when it's lacking in antioxidants, it adds continuously to the toxic burden. Most oxidative stress in the body is generated by cellular respiration, if you remember your biology class."

"Oh yes. The famous Krebs Cycle. Isn't the body equipped to do its own cleanup?"

"In most cases yes. There are endogenous enzymes and innate antioxidants responsible for detoxification. But without a regular supply of antioxidants, they get overwhelmed quickly. As you probably know, free radicals are unpaired electrons. In their search to neutralize themselves, they'll steal electrons from stable molecules, creating a cascade of more unpaired electrons."

"Can we take a pill to neutralize these raging free radicals?"

"You can, but it's not as effective as the antioxidants that come from food. You also have to reduce oxidative stress by adopting a clean diet."

"How do you reduce oxidative stress?"

His eyelids twitch for a second. He breathes deep before answering. "By consuming less of the foods that lack antioxidants. Having a healthy digestive system and reducing infections and stress are all helpful in lowering oxidation."

He stands and grabs a book with a white cover, boasting a bouquet of vibrant fruits and vegetables overflowing from a basket. The title, in golden yellow, jumps off the cover: *The Neglected Cure*.

"This is written by a scientist and contains a lot of information, with supporting evidence, establishing a direct link between meat consumption, diets poor in antioxidants, and the development of many diseases." He studies my face for a reaction as he puts the book in my hands.

"Are you vegan?" I ask sheepishly.

"We prefer to call the diet MicroRiche. It looks vegan because we remove all the animal products. But the diet is based on a simple biochemistry formula that increases the intake of micronutrients and antioxidants while lowering the amount of macronutrients. One thing to remember, Annie, is food does not make you a good or a bad person. It only affects your health."

I untangle my fingers with relief. "I'm glad to hear that."

He clearly knows how to earn a person's trust and change perspectives. "Do I have to eat this way for the rest of my life?"

"Let's have this conversation in three months, before you leave." He hands me a sterile plastic cup for urine collection. "We should get the results in a week or so, then we'll know more about your metabolism and the level of toxicity, if any."

"For your treatment plan, you'll receive weekly megadoses of vitamin C intravenously. You need to do a juice fast twice a week and take all the supplements Karina recommends."

"I heard large doses of vitamin C cause GI problems."

"Not when administered intravenously. We will be monitoring your symptoms and we will adjust the dose accordingly."

"How do yoga and meditation figure into all this?"

A soft laugh illuminates his face—a sign he's heard the question before. "Meditation is just another method of relaxation. Yoga is a good exercise. As you can see, there isn't a lot to do around here in this heat. You don't have to participate if you can find something better to do."

"I think I'll enjoy yoga, but meditation will either bore me to tears or put me to sleep."

As I leave his office, a heat wave rises in my chest, fanning the dim light of hope.

On the way back to my room, I stop by the kitchen for a drink of water. Stefani and Sonia are putting the last touches on a buffet of desserts—the Monday ritual mentioned in the brochure.

They've arranged three types of ice cream bowls on top of buckets of ice: matcha, chocolate, and vanilla next to a boat of chocolate sauce and a bowl of yogurt with yellow fruit pulp and brown seeds. I ask Sonia what type of fruit pulp it is, and she replies, *"Es maracujá!"* She grabs a fruit from the basket to show me—a purplish-brown round shell the size of a golf ball with dents that make it look old. I still can't identify it, so I pull out my cell phone and click on Google. The translator renders *passion fruit.*

Donna walks in. "Damn, I love matcha ice cream, but I'm fasting today." She squeezes her bottle of water and flees.

Marta, a thin blonde woman in her fifties with turquoise blue eyes, sits next to me. Her left arm is bigger than her right and is covered with a beige sleeve. Our ice cream trays are identical: samples of each flavor.

She wipes her chin before gushing about the desserts. “Here I thought vegan was ascetic. The chef actually grinds raw cocoa nibs into powder and mixes it with almond milk she makes herself.”

My spoon slides smoothly into the creamy texture, “I didn’t know coconut flesh could ferment into yogurt. I wonder if I could find the same in stores back home.”

“It won’t be this good. I mean, she made it two or three days ago,” says Marta.

The ice cream is made with different nut milks, date, or agave nectar as sweeteners, then flavored. The taste is more dense than regular ice cream. The vanilla has a sweet fragrance, unlike the pungent one in my usual store-bought pint. The grassy taste in the matcha ice cream is reminiscent of a freshly mowed lawn; the chocolate is so intense I can only eat a couple of spoonfuls.

“Do you really think they can heal us with this food?” I ask.

“It beats getting lymphedema.” Marta points to her chest, “When a new tumor sprang in my right breast ten years after the left one was removed, I told them ‘only surgery’ and made the surgeon promise not to remove any lymph nodes. I'd rather die from cancer than have another swollen arm.”

“Is your lymphedema under control?”

“As long as I nurture it. I have to wash these sleeves daily. They have to be replaced every six months. I also use a pump, which I did not bring here.” She sighs and fills her mouth with vanilla ice cream.

Marta has been at AM for two months. Aside from missing her dog and her family, it’s the best trip she’s ever taken. She glances over her swollen arm, imprisoned in level three compression. “I’ve learned so much about nutrition and what healthy cooking means. I’ll never go back to my old diet.” She swipes a hand over her belly. “I lost seven KILOS I’ve been carrying around since… I can’t even remember."

"Congratulations."

She grins. "Who knew we could put cancer in remission and lose weight with delicious food!"

"You make this place sound like Fatima."

"Prayers are not always answered, but food always delivers."

"Or is delivered." We laugh and Marta points her spoon at me. "Don't forget to attend the classes. Dr. Hidalgo and Karina are amazing."

Back in my room, I check my email and a message from my father comes with an attachment. After my diagnosis, he's been studying every article published on anaplastic astrocytoma. He sent me several articles about people who put cancer in remission with nutrition and holistic treatments. All anecdotal accounts. But modern medicine started with natural remedies, going back to the Greeks.

My video date with Daniel is in thirty minutes. I open my makeup case filled with powders, pencils, concealers, and lipsticks, then close it. It's silly to wear so much disguise for a video. I put on a light pink tank top, brush my hair, and turn on the camera.

He shows up twenty minutes late. A frown links his eyebrows and he looks more at his desk than at the camera.

"I'm sorry. Some family thing came up. How are you?" He puts on a forced smile, then raises his gaze. "You look radiant."

"Honey, what happened?"

"It's all good now. How did your meeting with the doctor go?"

"Is Tanya okay?"

"She's fine."

"Did you have to take her shopping?"

He lifts his chin, meeting my eyes. "I had to take Nina to the hospital."

"I'm so sorry. What happened?"

He swipes his hair back. "They'll keep her for a couple of

days, but she's stable."

Before I move to the next question, he's back to my medical encounter. So, I tell him about the judgmental nutritionist, the sweet doctor, the funny Ernesto, and my newfound love for vegan food. He softens his shoulders and sinks a little more into the chair.

"These people believe they can cure cancer with vegetables." I wave the *Neglected Cure* book in front of the camera.

"My grandmother used to say, when someone hands you a string of hope, weave it into a rope."

"Whatever you say. I'm stuck here for three months. Then I'll come after you for retribution."

He shakes his head with another paternalistic glare.

I have never seen him so preoccupied. Nina's situation must be more serious than he's letting on. In the absence of physical contact, I use humor to distract him.

"I learned a new word today: m*aracuja.*"

"*Maracuya*!" he replies with a scolding tone.

"It's cuter in Portuguese."

"I want you to learn Spanish, not the neighbor's language," he says with a stern voice, trying to hold back a laugh.

"The neighbor? You can't even say Brazil?"

"I'll learn their name when they learn to play football without cheating."

"Hey, they have great soccer players in Brazil."

"What kind of propaganda have you been listening to?"

I laugh until tears fill my eyes.

"I'm being facetious, but the rivalry between the two teams is real," he says.

"OK, *tu eres mi maracuya*. How's that for learning Spanish?"

"Estoy loco con contento."

"You sound so sexy when you speak Spanish."

"Hmm, been sexy all my life."

After we end our session, I stare at the computer screen

for several minutes, light and empty like autumn leaves in the wind. The inability to touch him, his reluctance to confide in me, all underline the multi-faceted isolation: I'm both cast out and caged in.

Walking to the dining room for a glass of kombucha, I run into Donna. With our beverages in hand, we sit by the pool. The psychologist in me takes over as I listen to her story. She came to the center three weeks ago. She's been suffering from fibromyalgia for years. Her husband moved out while she was in a hospital recovering from gallbladder surgery. He left his lawyer's business card stapled to an apologetic note for falling in love with someone else.

"I was actually relieved when he left." She gazes at the stars in the clear sky. "He was constantly putting me down and complaining. I just didn't have the strength to fight him. So, I stayed in bed most of the time and ate. Result: thirty pounds." She laughs and pulls on a roll of belly fat.

"It doesn't bother you that he left for another woman?"

She smirks. "Honey, she can have'm. She'll never get laid! He's been impotent for years." We chortle.

"How about Viagra?"

"He has so many allergies, he's scared of medication." She pauses and pulls her hair back. "When I get out of here, if I'm as healthy as they tell me I will be, I want to start a new business."

"Doing what?"

"I don't know... something in health. I've learned so much here and I realize so many diseases are food-related."

Donna has no fear or regrets. She's eager to jump into the future. Instead of counseling her, I'm the one being counseled. I need to be more patient with Daniel. He's in an awkward position. Far from pushing me away, he tries to carve a space for the two of us. With so many roadblocks in our way, if our relationship is to last, we have to hold on tight.

ΛΛΛ

I created a routine that keeps me busy while learning a new way to eat. Between the cooking classes, yoga, video dates with Daniel and my parents, and chatting with friends on social media, I've no time left for boredom. The bag of books I brought with me is still unopened. Only Robert, Tina, and Janet know the truth. Most people are envious of my sabbatical.

I revert into a counselor when I'm around other patients. I enjoy listening to their stories in the most intimate details. Sick people lose all inhibition and vulnerability. They talk freely about their illness, their fears, and their unwavering hope. More than the imminent threat of death, we all share one common trait: a determination to win. If this is our only option to beat cancer, then it will work. No other outcome is acceptable. I'm the only one who's still skeptical, but listening to story after story of the most desperate cases who have made a complete recovery, hope becomes contagious.

At every meal, the seven of us sit at the dining table by the pool, unmasked, surrounded by palm trees and cacti, sheltered from the blazing sun. If the food does not cure us, the setting probably will. As I chew each bite and listen to them talk, I often forget where I am and surrender to the vacation atmosphere.

/\ /\ /\

Karina says cooking is chemistry. Matching ingredients to create delicious meals is part art and part engineering. And she excels in both.

"By the time you leave Años Mejores, you will not only cook, you will enjoy it," she says, waving a whisk. "Once you understand food combining and seasoning, you can create innovative recipes as flavorful as the conventional dishes. You will dazzle your friends with your creations."

Donna whispers in my ear, "Let's not get carried away." I reply with a chuckle.

Karina pairs each class with a theme. There is one on cheese and yogurt, made with nuts, seeds, spices, and plant-derived thickeners such as Irish moss or agar agar— the famous vegan gelatin extracted from seaweed. She makes ricotta cheese from macadamia nuts and cashews and bakes a lasagna. It does taste like lasagna—just without meat.

Another class is all about burgers and how to replace old favorites. She creates turkey cutlets with chickpea flour and a special blend of seasonings.

"Burgers can be raw or cooked," says Karina as she forms perfectly round patties.

"A vegan steak tartar?" Ernesto teases.

She gives him a dirty look. In a food processor, she grinds sunflower seeds, chia and flax seeds, and sun-dried tomatoes into a meat-like mixture. Adding chopped yellow bell peppers, onions, and spices forms what she calls sun burgers. In addition to tasting good, they take minutes to assemble. I catch myself thinking *I can do this.*

Her cooked burgers don't disappoint either: beet burgers, bean burgers, harvest burgers—made with whole grain, mushrooms, nutritional yeast, and miso—and my favorite, which she names *le California*, made with lentils, olives, and walnuts. Her masterpiece, however, is "tuna". She blends forest cucumber, pumpkin seeds, onions, and seasonings. She flattens the mixture and shapes pieces resembling sushi and circulates a platter for us to sample.

"Doesn't it taste like tuna?" She proudly watches us inhale the entire dish with our gleaming faces.

We all admire Karina. Her passion for food is unmatched. In the kitchen, she's no longer imperious or fastidious. When someone asks a question, she beams and patiently explains how different ingredients combine to create unexpected flavors and textures. She lifts a bottle of pomegranate molasses and lists its health benefits before adding some to a pot of beans cooked with walnuts, cumin, and cilantro. "The tangy flavor of the thick syrup tickles the beans and boosts their taste."

Donna asks, "Is pomegranate juice a good source of antioxidants?"

"No, the juice you buy in the store is pasteurized and has water added. It's mainly liquid sugar," Karina replies. "In this recipe, the cooking process destroys the vitamins and antioxidants, but not the minerals. Iron, calcium, zinc, and magnesium are still there."

ΛΛΛ

Usually, my waking hour is regulated by the sun. Today, I wake before it. I spent the night waiting for the day to rise to prepare for Daniel's visit. Seeing a familiar face is something we all long for in this cocoon, away from civilization. COVID restrictions and the remoteness of the location make visitors a luxury. Through his connections, Daniel managed to obtain permission to see me every other week by presenting a negative PCR test and answering a questionnaire each time.

He won't be here until lunchtime, but I still rise early with the anticipation of a child waiting for a parent who comes home after a long absence. I try on several outfits, veto everything, and start over. I want to look cheerful. The only thing I can offer him is high-quality time when we're together.

For the first time, I opt for no makeup. I chose a long floral print dress. The lavender background is smeared with large white flowers against blue and pink swirls and a touch of green acting as leaves. I'll accessorize it with a large pink belt to give myself a sexy, yet elegant allure.

After breakfast, I walk along the Paseo de la Serenidad. Birds flit and flirt with each other in the trees, under the timid early morning sun. The Hill of Seven Colors looks a lot closer from this side of the compound. I wonder what the view from the top would be like.

It's only 9:00 a.m. when I return to my room. I shower, dress, and rush to the phone—two more hours to go.

Around 11:30, WhatsApp announces his arrival. I open the door and he's already behind it. He enters and scans me head to toe before hugging me.

"You look beautiful and refreshed. Your face has more pink in it now."

"I think it's the Argentinian heat."

We sit on the bed, his arm around me while I rest my head on his shoulder. All is peaceful and quiet, as if the Earth stopped spinning after reaching a destination. He plays with my fingers. I want to stay here, suspended in the sweet emotion of his presence, but I feel a compulsion to talk, a need to know more about his life—the one he lives without me. I need the small details missing on video. Those ordinary life details that would bridge the distance between us.

"How's Nina?"

He sighs and looks down at his shoes before answering. "Not good."

"What's wrong?"

"She can't breathe well. She's gotten all kinds of infections. She's better now, but the doctors are not optimistic."

"I'm so sorry. How is Tanya?"

"I haven't told her anything. I want her to enjoy her time with her mother the best she can."

He pulls away from me. "Let's go to lunch and try this food you've been raving about."

"Daniel, let me be there for you."

"I want this weekend to be about you."

"It's been about me for quite some time. I can't do much from here, but I can listen and offer support."

"You're going to charge me for counseling, aren't you?"

"You can't afford me." I giggle and he kisses me to avoid further questions.

We step outside the dark cloud by putting everything aside Nina's fragile state, my cancer, and the physical distance that separates us. We leap into a present where we exist as a happy couple—for a limited time.

6 - The Other Woman

I wake up before daybreak and curl on the bed, chin on knees, arms wrapped around bent legs. In just a few hours, I will learn how my body works and maybe why it's become a breeding ground for tumors. What if some gene mutation will keep the tumor growing? What if AM can't help me? I churn negative thoughts like a drowning woman staring at the sun above water.

I robotically check my online calendar—a white sheet divided into blank squares. Next Saturday, the twentieth of February, I turn thirty-nine, possibly my last birthday. But that's not the worst of it. Lying in a hospital bed, disfigured, drooling, and spitting word salad is what dominates my fears.

I close the browser and lift my head to watch the dust particles dance in the sunbeams pouring through the window. Maybe I'll get lucky. The tumor might push on the nerves and provoke a seizure, which will ease the transition from life to *eternal peace.*

I plunge a heating rod into a mug of water to brew a cup of tea, then make the bed before heading out to breakfast. This little room has become home, so I tidy up daily and put the laundry in a box under the bed. Once the box is full, I take it to Stefani or Sonia for washing. It's a reduced life, but slowly becoming comfortable.

On the way to breakfast, I lose my appetite. I grab another cup of tea and I'm about to leave when Donna walks in.

"No breakfast this morning?"

"I have an appointment with Dr. Hidalgo. My stomach is tied in knots."

"Ah, your toxicity test!" She pushes her hair back on her shoulders, sets her plate on the edge of the buffet, and points at me with a spoon. "Don't let him throw all that bio-chem mumbo jumbo at you."

"I'm more concerned about what the test will reveal."

"You'll be fine. It's just a sneak peek into what your cells are doing. Mine were plain lazy." She hands me a small bowl.

"At least have some yogurt with granola. It's divine."

I obey and try the coconut yogurt topped with granola. After a couple of spoonfuls, my stomach locks.

Dr. Hidalgo waits for me in the dark office with his usual soft smile. Today, he's wearing a suit and tie and looks a little taller. He pulls a chair next to him for me to sit and review the test results together. His hand rests on a small stack of papers in the middle of the desk, and he opens the first set. Each page is lined with multicolor horizontal bars, each representing a metabolite. The bars are displayed in three color gradients: green for good, yellow for borderline, and red for what needs fixing. A black diamond is positioned on each line to indicate the level of the metabolite.

His warm and peaceful presence fills me with a warm sensation that relaxes me like a child who sees his mother after a long absence. I listen to his words as I breathe in the lavender aroma permeating the office.

"Annie, don't be apprehensive. These are just findings. Whatever issue we find, we can fix. We just want to make sure all your nutrients are balanced and all the detoxification pathways are clear, and your body has the required cofactors to maximize your results during your stay here."

The first page we look at is about methylation.

"Your vitamin B12 and folate levels are near perfect, which means there's nothing wrong with your methylation cycle."

"I can use some good news."

"I always start with these two nutrients because a lot of people have a gene mutation called MTHFr that interferes with the metabolism of these vitamins, but they're unaware of it because conventional medicine does not do these types of tests." He turns to the next page.

"If you have been feeling depressed lately or agitated…"

"I've felt a lot of that, but it was before coming here. Let me tell you, I was not pleasant to be around."

He smiles and puts his hand on my shoulder. "That explains the low level of serotonin. Either you're not synthesizing enough or it's used up. But this is due to stress, not cancer."

I nod, cross my arms over my chest, and continue studying the results.

He turns the page to the famous Krebs cycle. The little black diamonds are all over the place. Some markers are high, others low, with very few in the normal range. He points at some biochemistry words— adipate, ethylmalonate— and says that, when these are high, it means my fat metabolism is impaired. My carbohydrate metabolism is no better, and neither is my amino acid catabolism. He shows me another picture that illustrates these energy pathways and their required nutrients at each stage. All my nutrients are diverted to repair and detoxification in the post-surgery phase.

"So, this chronic fatigue will get better?"

"Correct. It's due to nutrient depletion. You should feel more energetic in two to three weeks."

A liver diagram lists all the nutrients needed for detoxification. So many vitamins and minerals are required to run this small factory. Dr. Hidalgo talks about biochemistry the same way a poet talks about love. His speech flows like the calming current of a brook in the spring. He reminds me of my father when he talks about plants, their families, their genetics, and how they communicate. If he never mentioned the word plant, one would think he was talking about some human tribe.

Dr. Hidalgo points at a long name abbreviated as 8-OHdG. His happy and flirty disposition changes into a more serious tone. He stares at the sheet of paper as he delivers the news.

"You see this marker? It's very high. This is oxidative stress that damages DNA. It's also implicated in the cause of cancer, diabetes, and other degenerative diseases."

"Can something be done about it?"

"Of course. You need a lot of antioxidants, particularly vitamin C. But you're also depleted of other nutrients that need to be replenished."

I point at the diamond anchored on the red part of the assessment bar. "What causes this marker to go up so high?"

"It's a variety of factors. Pollution, smoking for some people, medication, infections, or just a lack of antioxidants."

He pauses to study my reaction. I breathe deep and nod.

"You see, conventional medicine focuses on the symptom of a single item. They rarely take into account other low-level effects of multiple toxins until they accumulate into a burden that leads to disease. Then they treat the disease, but never consider its origin."

"What would've happened if I had taken chemo?"

"You would be poisoned further. You'd feel more tired and would take longer to recover, in addition to all the symptoms caused by the side effects. It's a violent treatment that affects all cells in your body, but is most taxing to the liver, which is in charge of cleaning up the byproducts of chemicals."

"And no guarantee of success."

"That's true for any treatment. But the problem is, after chemotherapy, they never tell you what to do to return your body to good health. The side effects of chemotherapy can linger for months. Other side effects can manifest years after treatment."

"What kind of side effects?"

"It's totally random. We had a lady who was treated for five years. She developed allergies to most plant foods. Another patient had breast enlargement."

He purses his lips and frowns. "We get people here who've been intoxicated by medication alone for years. They take yet another medication to counteract the side effects of the first one. Their bodies turn into chemical plants, their liver barely functioning. Within three weeks in this place, they feel alive again. After three months, many leave completely healed."

"How come none of this is covered in the media? Why isn't the medical community investigating nutrition?"

A smirk is painted on his face. "What's in it for them?" He turns the page and stops. "If people took better care of themselves and ate healthy, the pharmaceutical industry would lose billions. But don't get me wrong, there is a place for medication. Painkillers are a wonderful invention."

He turns another page and he's cheerful again. I have no heavy metal accumulation and no dysbiosis.

He puts the test results in a folder and pushes it toward me. "This is your copy. Review the results and my notes and let me know if you have any questions." He opens another folder filled with brochures and a treatment plan.

"Your first injection of vitamin C is already planned for tomorrow. You will also start a juice fast twice a week."

An involuntary grimace curls my lips downward.

"The juices taste good and you shouldn't feel too hungry. You will find all the recipes and their ingredients in this booklet. If there is a vegetable you're averse to, just let the kitchen know and they'll customize it for you."

"Two days every week?"

He chuckles. "After a couple of times, you'll enjoy fasting. Talk to Donna. She was the most resistant. Now, she loves it."

"I'm not the only one you want to torture?"

"We hurt everyone equally." His beautiful brown eyes light up when he laughs, and dimples form on his cheeks.

I stand to leave and he makes one step forward as if he wants to hug me, but stops himself when I look away, tucking the folder under my arm. I walk to my room with renewed confidence and make a mental list of all the things I'll share with my Dad at our next video meeting. Outside, the sun pours its flaming rays on the land.

I enter the room, put the folder on the table and check WhatsApp. I'm interrupted by a knock on the door.

Donna comes to check on me. "How did your meeting go?"

"I learned a lot. He wants me to fast. *Starting tomorrow!*"

"You'll get used to it," she says, plopping herself on the

only chair in the room. "The first day was so hard I almost went to the recreation room to eat when nobody was watching. But after the third time, I didn't feel the urge to eat as much. I can fast for weeks now. I feel so good afterward, but you don't have my problem."

She picks up the picture frame on the little table under the window and examines it. The picture was taken at the Auberge des Assassins—my first date with Daniel. He's standing behind me with his arm across my chest. It's the only decoration in my minimalist living quarters.

"Is this your boyfriend? He's gorgeous. I only got a glimpse of him when he came to visit. I was fasting that day, so I stayed in my room." She pauses. "Is he good to you? Argentinian men are flakey."

"Not this one," I reply, my back turned to her.

"That's what they all say. Make sure he's not snacking on the side."

"He's very loyal. I've never been this happy with a man."

As I tell her about my relationship, her eyes shine and her grin grows bigger. "I'm so happy for you. How long have you been seeing each other? Any wedding bells on the horizon?"

"It's a new relationship, no wedding plans."

"Where did you meet him?"

"On a scuba diving trip."

"Ah… That's what I need, but I'm too fat. I'd frighten the fish."

"You're weightless in the water and everyone looks alike. You don't have to worry about your hair, nails—"

"Then I should live there, not just visit. Change my name to Cousteau."

"You'll lose the weight. Especially if they're starving us."

Donna reflects for a moment. "I just want to feel good. I've been bedridden for six years. The meds didn't work alone and made me sicker when combined. At forty-eight, I felt eighty-eight."

Dr. Hidalgo's words echo in my head as Donna describes

her pain. I wonder how many people suffer from unexplained symptoms that can be fixed with a simple tweak of biochemistry and veggies.

"But why are *you* here? You're young, thin, beautiful. Do you have cancer?"

Donna always asks direct questions. She has the curiosity of a detective and the mind of a journalist. Her candor forces me to face the new reality. I'm a patient in this place.

"I have a brain tumor. My prognosis is not so good. I was told I have less than a year to live."

Donna stares at me in disbelief. Her mouth opens, but she makes no sound. Cancer generates an awkward discomfort. She quickly regains her composure. "Don't believe the medical pricks. You can beat it. People do it all the time. You're in good hands here."

We smile. Neither of us may be entirely convinced that AM can cure me, but it doesn't hurt to hope.

"You know, when I told my doctor I was in pain, I mean, I was hurting all over. My fingers looked like hotdogs; my face was as puffy as a marshmallow. Do you know what the prick said?"

"You needed an antidepressant?"

"He told me to lose weight. I was so mad, I told him to fuck off. He called security to escort me out. I got in my car and cried all the way home."

"There are so many diseases that medicine doesn't understand yet. Unfortunately, some doctors won't admit it. I'm sorry you suffered so much."

"I'm starting to feel better, though. Yesterday, I walked the entire Paseo de whatever out there. Haven't been able to walk more than a few steps for years."

I put my arm around her shoulders. "Come on, let's go to lunch. I'm fasting tomorrow. I need to store up."

Once again, the lunch buffet is a feast for all the senses. A large flower arrangement anchors the back of the buffet, with a jug of fresh water on each side. Today is Raw Food Day. We gather around and read the names of the dishes and their ingredients before sampling them.

The meal starter is a cucumber soup served in a clay pot. The ingredients read mint, apple, and lime juice, and the soup is topped with diced mango and mint leaves.

Two large oval platters are piled with a colorful salad. The first one is called Complexity. It's a rainbow of colors from pineapple, red bell peppers, radishes, and pumpkin seeds on a bed of microgreens. The second one is more copious. Sprouted quinoa, cashews, sprouted lentils, and shaved radicchio are tossed in a citrus-maracuja coulis.

For dessert, we are treated to chocolate mousse. Cocoa nibs ground to powder, mixed with coconut milk, whipped with honey, and served with raw raspberry jam. We all agree the dessert is a transcendent experience but a bit heavy. Pablo takes only two bites of his ramekin. Ernesto doesn't care for chocolate, but Donna, Anna-Magdalena, and I clean our ramekins.

We sit by the pool, and everyone shares their travel stories. They chat and laugh as if life is normal for all of us. Nobody complains. Occasionally, someone mentions missing a family member or their pet, but we all try to live in defiance of disease, inside a bubble, suspended in space and time.

Ernesto asks about Daniel, whom he calls El Porteño. Then he tells me about his family and how much he misses working. His eyes travel beyond the pool, where two butterflies are fighting over a flower.

"How about hobbies? Things you do for fun?" I ask.

"Everything I do is to improve life for my family."

"Can you think of something that would give you joy without being useful?"

He twists his head as if he wants to wring out a thought. "I like to bike."

He launches into a long description of what he enjoys about biking and his face lights up as he elaborates on the beauty of nature. The solitude of riding deep into the woods, climbing hills, and exploring areas where cars can't go.

Different fragrances from flowers, leaves, mushrooms, and decaying plants all form a warm blanket that fosters a world of insects.

“Maybe I will do some biking when I go back. Annie, do you know what’s best thing about biking?”

“Fresh air, exercise?”

“Yes… But most important, wife cannot… how to say in English…”

“Nag?”

“Yes, no wife.”

“She doesn’t like biking?”

“Doesn’t know how.”He laughs and tilts his head back, exposing his Adam's apple. Beneath the layers of years and hardship is a handsome man.

“When you go back home, I want you to bike again, okay?”

He turns to me, as if a lightbulb switched on in his head. "Annie, this is the best idea I've had in long time. Well, your idea."

"Credit is irrelevant. As long as you take some time for relaxation and do the things you enjoy. Believe it or not, exercise, recreational activities, and spending time with family and friends all contribute to fostering good health."

After lunch, I rush to my room for a video date with my parents. Many patients sleep in the afternoon. I napped every day during my first two weeks. Then one day, I was without fatigue.

My mother is the first to come on video.

“You look beautiful and rested. I need to try this place.”

“You should see the food. We have to learn to cook this way, Mom.”

“I hope you’re eating enough. You need to gain some weight. Your face is still gaunt. Do you sleep well? How is the fatigue?"

"I sleep very well, eight hours most nights. I don't remember ever having this much energy. If it weren't for the yoga class, I'd be jumping off the walls."

I get misty-eyed when my father starts talking. Video is like seeing someone on the other side of the road; we can wave, talk, and smile, but no intimate conversations, no hugs, and I so miss his warmth and reassurance when he puts his arms around me and squeezes my shoulders. He often remarks how I'm taller than him.

The pandemic has taken a toll on both my parents. My mother is more withdrawn and stopped dying her white hair, which outlines the wrinkles on her face. My father looks aged, too, and tired. Even through the video, I see he's paler and his cheeks sag a little.

"Mom, you need to dye your hair. You're starting to look like Mark Twain."

"I'm saving money for a facelift."

"You don't need a facelift!" My father sneers. "You need your head examined. Here's your new patient, Annie."

"Sorry, I don't work with friends or family."

For once in a long time, there's no mention of cancer. Our conversation flows as usual—Mother's encoded messages of love, Father offering his wisdom, and me making fun of everything.

Λ Λ Λ

I open the folder Dr. Hidalgo gave me and pull out the fasting schedule.

Your fasting days are Mondays and Thursdays for ten weeks.

One serving of juice four times a day. Please drink plenty of water between each juice serving. Juices will vary in sweetness and bitterness, depending on the ingredients used. Feel free to add fizzy water or a squeeze of lemon to make them more enjoyable.

At 8:00 a.m., Stefani knocks on my door with a tray of green juices that look like stagnant water from somewhere in a dark forest. The accompanying note says *dandelion leaves, celery, basil, lime, pineapple*. My stomach screams *NO* and my lips seal shut.

I put the small glasses on the table next to the picture frame while I assemble the courage to drink the green substance. I lift the first glass, close my eyes, and down the content into two giant gulps. I move to the second one and empty it as well. I save the last one for later—after I recover from the first two. Far from delicious, but not as bad as I expected.

/\ /\ /\

After yoga, we assemble in the recreation room for Dr. Hidalgo's nutrition class. I'm eyeing the snacks and fruit basket. New to fasting, my desire to eat stems more from fear of hunger than hunger itself.

Donna is also fasting and when she catches me staring at the food, she rolls her eyes. "You'll get used to it, hon."

Dr. Hidalgo enters the room carrying a laptop case and a fat folder under his arm. After he greets us, he plugs the computer into the television and starts a PowerPoint presentation. His slight frame, enveloped in a crisp white shirt with a black belt and black trousers, disappears in the large bookcase behind him. As soon as he speaks, his voice is drowned by the ear-splitting jackhammers strafing the pavement outside. He apologizes for the noise and proceeds with his lecture.

Today, we learn about the microbiome. He covers the role of fiber in the diet and how it serves as food for the microbiota, which make vitamins. His eyes lock with mine when he discusses the HPA axis and the brain-gut communication. He's more versed in brain biochemistry than I am—the necessary nutrients and the enzymes required to break them down and synthesize hormones. I never gave much thought to the nutrition aspect of mental health.

Without saying the word "meat," he dives into the long list of health problems caused by a high-protein diet. His PowerPoint slide titles are straight to the point. *Paleo: when life was brutish and short*; Ketogenic *Diet: how to pickle your liver. Vegetarian: the hypocrite's diet.* Everyone laughs. Ernesto raises his hand.

"The food we eat here is vegetarian. Is that no good?"

"So-called vegetarians eat eggs and milk products. Eggs, cheese, and their derivatives are high in saturated fat and cholesterol. These foods can increase the risk of diabetes and inflammation, not to mention weight gain. The diet we have here at Años Mejores is called Microriche. We don't use any foods that contain saturated fat. The food is naturally high in micronutrients, fiber, and antioxidants, yet low in fat, carbohydrates, and proteins." He surveys our reaction, then adds, "You heard that right, low in proteins."

A few people in the audience look lost when he covers the ins and outs of protein composition—their function and how they're metabolized in the body— and shocked by the revelation that excess protein does more harm than good. I always thought the more the better when it came to protein. But he says animal products are high in an amino acid called phenylalanine which competes with tryptophan for absorption in the brain. A depletion in tryptophan leads to a deficiency in serotonin, the feel-good hormone. Depression and mood swings can follow. His tone becomes serious and almost emphatic when he lists all the deleterious effects of a high-protein diet on human health. His voice increases by a few octaves when he refutes their credibility.

He clears his throat and points a finger at the screen. "None of these diets is supported by science or created by a nutrition scientist."

Donna and I look at each other and share a guilty smile. We know he's talking about us. Nonetheless, he provides sound scientific evidence to support his claims, which motivates me to read the book he gave me at our first meeting.

Before we leave, he opens the folder and hands each of us a questionnaire. He wants us to answer the questions and bring them back to the next session for discussion.

Glancing at the questions, I whisper to Donna, "I think we're getting indoctrinated."

After we leave the presentation, Donna and I sit around the pool and hope the scenery will make fasting more tolerable.

She says, "I think Dr. Hidalgo likes you. He was constantly looking in your direction."

"He does not! He was looking at both of us because we're the biggest meat eaters in the group."

"Then why was he staring at your legs?"

"Are you a soap opera writer in Hollywood?"We giggle like schoolgirls.

"He's cute. If I were as hot as you, I'd hit on him."

"Maybe he wants to hit on you, but he's too professional."

"Yeah, maybe he'll use me as alien repellent."

"Alien what?"

"Alien repellent. When aliens see me from space, they don't land."

Donna is constantly self-deprecating. She's hurting and resents the changes in her body. Her beautiful figure is distorted by a sagging belly. Her face sags a little, too, now that all the puffiness is gone. She always laughs at herself as if to prevent others from doing so. But her beauty is still there. She has luxurious blonde hair she wears long and wild; she always wears unicolor dresses accented with a contrasting colorful scarf she lets hang down to her knees. Her smile can be seen miles away.

"Donna, you need to say kind things about your body. What comes out of your mouth becomes your reality."

"Annie? Cut it out. I want you to be my friend, not my therapist. I look like shit. I feel even worse. You have a hard time adjusting to being a patient. I can't adjust to being ugly and out of shape. Do you know I used to be a model? A COO with twelve managers and directors reporting to me?"

"When did the weight go up?"

"When I turned forty. I thought it was from being

overworked and eating in restaurants all the time. As a COO of a large corporation, you don't get to cook. You're lucky if you make your own coffee."

"You could've hired a personal chef."

"Another employee to manage! Dr. Hidalgo says I have mitochondrial insufficiency and a defective digestive system, so I was malnourished and had food allergies, and it just snowballed from there. So, besides starvation, they're doping me with supplements. As much as I hate giving up bacon, I have to say I feel better than I have in years."

"Did you confess to eating bacon?"

"Yeeeesss, and Karina said there will be no forgiveness. Hell is my destination."

We share a resounding laugh; Sonia and Stefani look in our direction.

Donna continues."You know, these people are on to something. All the doctors I've seen just told me to go on a low-carb diet and lose weight. The more I tried those diets, the sicker I got. But I lost twelve pounds in just a month on this diet and I can walk a mile without rest or being out of breath."

"See, it's just a matter of time before you get your model figure back."

"So, what're *your* plans after you leave this place?"

Her question hits me like a slap across the face. Returning home means getting a final answer. That moment when this thread of hope I've been hanging onto might break into shreds. It's a terrifying stage of thought I don't want to enter.

I ask, "Do you believe in dreams?"

She squints and brushes a tussock of hair behind her ear. "You mean like a prince will kiss me and I'll live happily ever after? Where's that bastard?"

"No, I mean dreams, like when you sleep."

"Only when they're good."

"I was dreaming of being in a small, dark tunnel with a friend. It was all black, like old dried lava. Spikes of black stones protruded everywhere, like upside down icicles. I was following my friend. She was small and had the stature of a child, but I couldn't see her face. The tunnel was so narrow we walked on our knees, poked by the stone spears. Then we reached the end of the tunnel and she jumped out and ran without waiting for me. I was to follow her because we were going to a New Year's Eve party. But when I wanted to exit the tunnel, there was a small wall I needed to jump over to catch up with my friend. As I contemplated how to jump, I woke up."

Donna frowns. "That's quite a dream."

"It means one of two things: either this will be over and there is a good life waiting for me, or the friend is an angel taking me to party with Jesus and Elvis."

We laugh and Donna looks at me with a motherly attitude. "You'll be okay, Annie. Many people put cancer in remission. This place would be closed down by now if they didn't deliver, you know?"

/\ /\ /\

My last juice is delivered at 6:00 p.m. The ingredients this time are cabbage, carrots, apples, turmeric, and ginger. It's slightly bitter and spicy. After I gulp it down, I brush my teeth to clean away the aftertaste. I comb my hair and put on a red sleeveless blouse before my video date with Daniel.

He logs in ahead of me, more cheerful than he's been in days. Sitting on a bench in the yard, he's stunning in a purple T-shirt. Nina's health is stable and they just celebrated Tanya's sixteenth birthday. He has made a selection of pictures to show me, which includes only those of Tanya, himself, and some random people. Each time I think of him in a family where I don't belong, the same twinge jabs at my gut. I was never the jealous or possessive kind, but the more hopeless I feel, the more I want to hold on to him. I want to dominate his thoughts, penetrate his life, so everything else is smaller. I become suddenly aware of the fragility of our relationship. If he had to make a choice, his family would come first. Instead of discouraging me, the "second position" fuels my desire to fight and gain more territory. It's silly, but feelings often are.

He's so proud of his daughter as a young woman, a gifted painter, and an A student. The more he sings her praises, the more distant I feel. I tell myself it's a different kind of love, but she's still number one. He sees a change in my demeanor and turns off the screen sharing. Embarrassed, I excuse myself to grab some water.

"It's cruel to show me pictures of food. Been fasting all day. Apparently, to cleanse my body of evil toxins."

He keeps his head down. Too late, he sensed my insecurities. "Annie, lo siento mucho, mi amor. It was insensitive of me to show you those pictures while you're going through so much. I just wanted you to see Tanya."

"No, I don't mind at all. Your daughter is beautiful and I'm glad you could celebrate her birthday. I just feel weak because of the fasting. I'm so hungry I can't think straight."

I'm not sure he's convinced, but he likes the explanation. I don't know how he can always see through me. I steer the conversation toward lighter topics. "Why does Ernesto call you El Porteño?"

"That's what the rest of the country calls those of us who live in Buenos Aires."

"Tu eres mi Porteño favorito."

"You're learning Spanish?"

"Whenever I'm bored, I fool around with some online classes. I'm not as tired as when I got here, so the more energy I have, the more bored I get."

"I'll be there Saturday. I'll help you use up some of that energy."

When he smiles, his whole face lights up, giving me a sense of peace—a feeling of forgiveness.

We exit the Zoom app on a positive note, but I feel like someone punched me in the gut. Three phrases echo in my head like one of those nightmare scenes in movies. *He's married; his family is number one; I'm the other woman.* The words get louder, then swirl around until I'm dizzy. I stretch on the bed, but my mind is flooded with images of him and Nina. I revisit Tanya's birthday pictures; she was standing next to him, kissing him, hugging him; The pride he expresses when he looks at her... I pull the sheet over my face, but the images are stubborn and refuse to fade.

I'm in uncharted territory without tools for navigation. I should be a source of comfort to a man dealing with a debilitated spouse and raising a teenager. But how can I do that when I'm sitting on the edge—invisible? Is it unreasonable to want more?

My mother never let me read fairy tales. She believes they're instruments to keep women weak and subservient. Consequently, I never dreamed of the savior prince, but I never thought I would be an actress in a poisoned love drama that's unlikely to end with happiness for all. Our love breeds in a bubble, detached from all things that make a conventional relationship. While most people envy romantic dinners or exotic getaways, I find myself fascinated by ordinary daily details. Every habitual life task such as grocery shopping, washing dishes, or celebrating a birthday becomes a special gesture with new dimensions when performed by someone you love with someone they love.

It's past 2:00 a.m. when I slide under the covers and turn off the bedside lamp. The room is bathed in a bright orange light. I look up and a harvest moon hangs in the sky surrounded by thousands of stars sprinkling the stark black sky. The high altitude brings the stars closer to the Earth; with the dryness of the desert and lack of pollution, nothing stands in the way of their little sparkles. I fall asleep gazing at the stars in the hours of tomorrow.

ΛΛΛ

It's Saturday and Daniel is on his way. I check the time and trace his itinerary online. His plane landed long ago;

he's probably about to arrive. I always get nervous when waiting for him. Every date is like the first, filled with the same excitement. Then I worry about how empty I'll feel the next day, watching him drive away, back to his life. After each visit, I need a few days to bounce back. All my hesitations fade away when a red car pulls into the driveway, in front of the reception office.

I race to the car. He steps out and removes his sunglasses, but the mask stays on. I throw my arms around him and we stay entwined under the quietness of the bright sunshine. His hair is shorter, and his skin has taken on a bronze color. As I breathe the fresh desert air and feel his breath on my neck, I float outside of my body and enter a world where all is beauty.

Donna runs towards us and, before I go through the introductions, she extends her hand and cheerfully announces, "You must be Daniel. I've heard a lot about you."

"And you are?"

"Oh, I'm Donna, Annie's friend. *Ahnshantay*."

"Pleased to meet you," Daniel says with a bow.

He's poised, elegant, and nice to my friend. After we enjoy a brief chat with Donna, he checks in at the reception desk and follows me to my room. As soon as the door closes, we hold each other and kiss—like any ordinary couple who's been together for years. We gently fall on the queen-size bed. We kiss some more. Then he puts his hand on my head and pulls away to look me in the eyes with his usual half smile. A question is coming.

"You freaked out when I showed you Tanya's pictures."

"I did?" My cheeks are inflamed and I'm sure turned red. I look away.

"Annie… I can love more than one person."

"I'm still the other woman!"

The words fly out of my mouth before I can think. I've been feeling so many things for so long that it all bubbles up to the surface and squirts out. I hyper-blink to repress welling tears.

"What would you like me to do?" he asks in a soothing voice.

I sit with my head turned to the wall and tersely reply, "I don't know!"

"Do you know what it would do to Tanya if I just walked away? What kind of example would that send to her?"

"I can only worry about myself right now!"

"Maybe it's time to grow up."

"What's that supposed to mean?"

"You always think only about yourself."

"Maybe because nobody else does!" I growl.

"Do you really mean that?"

I stare at my knees and regain my composure.

"Be careful, Annie," he says with that commanding voice again.

He's right. I'm acting like a child, but I need to vent. So much has been taken from me and I have to share the man I love. He sits next to me while I turn into my mother. Knees to chest, arms hugging legs, I suppress all emotions and become a ball of ice. "This is all new to me. I have a hard time adjusting to being number two—actually three."

"I didn't know there was a numbering system."

He clasps his hands and takes them to his forehead. Then he proceeds with what sounds like counseling but is actually a shaming speech. "True, my child comes first. Aside from that, I've been totally devoted to you—as much as distance allows. Once you're out of here, we can work out a solution, but you can't always have what you want when you want it."

After a long pause, he adds, "If you want to move on... I understand." His voice is low but loud enough to trigger an emotional avalanche within me.

"Now you wanna get rid of me?" I snap.

He bursts into laughter and pushes me to my side ."You're looking for a fight."

Before I answer, he opens my arms, pins them down, and kisses me. My anger is tamed by his touch and our closeness is restored. I have just learned the difference between love and want.

7 - A New Pair of Shoes

I flip through social media pictures of friends, reading their stories, political posts, and jokes. It's like looking in the rearview mirror of a slow-moving car. It's only been five weeks since I left my life, but every day pulls me farther from it and into a future I can't plan for or control. Perhaps the most difficult part of being sick is not knowing what tomorrow—if tomorrow... I live in a gray area, littered with maybe, hopefully, and similar adjectives that act as palliatives for the pain of waiting.

When I was eight, I developed a system to cope with my father's absence whenever he went on a business trip. Every morning I'd run to the calendar and X out the day. At night, I'd count how many days were left until his return. I dreamt of having superpowers to control time so I could speed through boring days, delete the bad ones, or dial back to happy times like birthdays and holidays. While those superpowers never manifested, I have retained the habit of counting days to get through tough times. So, I tally the days and watch the weeks decrease to reach my departure date.

Dad displays on my muted phone.

"Annie? Are you all right?"

"I don't know if I can do this, Dad."

"You want to leave? What happened?"

"I'm talking about my relationship. It's wrong on so many levels."

"Annie, get to the point."

"I had a fight with Daniel. This other woman thing is not for me."

"I was wondering how long it would take. It's not like you to be involved with a married man."

"He's been very good to me. Flying to see me every other weekend during a pandemic is not easy."

As much as I resent the situation, reminding me it's wrong is jarring and motivates me to hold on.

"I know. He's a good man in a bad situation. But you would be wasting your best years sharing him with someone else."

Why does it matter? The distance makes the "someone else" invisible; Cancer makes long-term plans futile.

"Any decision I make will result in a loss. But if I'm dying in a few months, the decision will be made by default."

"Do you realize what you're saying? You want to die so you don't have to deal with the situation? What's happening to you?"

"I'm not ready to let him go."

"There is no good time to end a relationship. We just choose when to hurt."

/\ /\ /\

The center abounds with creativity to keep us entertained. Every Friday, Chef Laora features another exotic cuisine. A vase with little green-and-yellow-striped flags with center stars serves as the centerpiece for the dining table. After greeting everyone with "Buenos dias, amigos," I ask what country we're celebrating. They answer "Senegal" in unison.

"Am I the only one who's flag-blind?"

"No, but perhaps the only one who can't read." Donna laughs and points at the card on the table, which reads "Senegal" in bold letters.

An oatmeal-like mixture of millet and coconut milk steams in a clay pot. It's sprinkled with cinnamon, topped with pumpkin seeds, and served with a side of yogurt, walnuts, and our usual birch syrup. An African basket, made of elephant grass and bright colors, holds slices of French baguette. Next to the bread is a bowl of sauce made with onions, chayote fruit, stewed tomatoes, and a casserole of jasmine rice with peanut sauce. The ingredients are all familiar—except millet—but the amazing flavors are new to most of us. Chef Laora and Karina combine ingredients the same way a painter combines colors. They can take the most boring vegetable, slice it, marinate it, season it, and sprinkle it with magic.

Diana arrives with two new patients. She introduces them as Claudette and Julie, mother and daughter from Belgium. Julie is on crutches and looks like a teenager. She avoids touching the ground as she stands. Diana leaves to let them partake in breakfast.

Everyone enjoys the meal and carries on like every morning. Julie and Claudette sit together outside the group. I can't help but wonder what disease afflicts this child.

Julie is thin, shy, and withdrawn. Her brown hair hangs on her shoulders with a few strands shading her eyes. Her face and neck are visibly swollen. She avoids eye contact. I introduce myself and talk to the mother.

"Julie has CRPS, Complex Regional Pain Syndrome," Claudette says between bites.

"I've never heard of it."

Claudette looks worn out. Her short black hair contrasts with her pale skin. Deep wrinkles vertically divide her cheeks; rosacea reddens the tip of her long nose. Her sorrow is palpable, but I sense a fierce determination to fight. She swallows and lifts her chin. "It's one of those orphan diseases. No one knows what causes it and there is no treatment. This is our last hope. We've seen every type of doctor under the sun."

"Bonjour, Julie," I gush, using the only French word I know.

She smiles and continues to chew on a piece of walnut without looking at me. I ask Claudette, "When was she diagnosed?"

"Five years ago. She was eighteen, and we were told she'll never walk again. She's a little better now after many therapies."

"They really perform miracles here."

Claudette smiles sideways and wrinkles her face. Her chin has an orange-peel texture. "That's what we were told. As much as I'd like to believe it, I'm hesitant to get my hopes up. We've hit so many dead ends already." She shakes her head in despair, then frowns and examines my face. "Are you one of the therapists here?"

"No, I'm a patient, but I'm a licensed psychologist. If you need to talk, I'm here to listen."

I excuse myself and run to my room to Google CRPS. The CRPS foundation site lists the disease as a neuro-inflammatory disorder. A malfunction of the nervous system which sends continuous pain signals to the brain. Although the cause is still unknown, CRPS occurs after a musculoskeletal or nerve injury. All the reputable sources cite the pain as being excruciating. I continue sifting through the information until I'm interrupted by a knock at the door. Claudette is my guest. I let her in and, after we exchange a few comments about Años Mejores she gets straight to the point. "I have a favor to ask. You say you're a psychologist. Do you think you could talk to Julie?"

"Sure. Will she let me?"

"You might be the best person to help her because you're also a patient. She's very withdrawn and shuts down when in public. At home, it's constant explosions of rage, which she alternates with crying. She already attempted to kill herself."

"Have you tried getting her into therapy at home?"

"She won't go. She's disillusioned with the whole medical system."

The memory of despair and hopelessness is still vivid. A shiver runs over my skin. "I can try."

"Of course, I'll pay for your time."

"That won't be necessary."

"I warn you, it won't be easy. She'll probably cuss at you in French or German."

"I won't take offense."

"She threw out Dr. Hidalgo."

"Why did she do that?"

"She's in constant pain. It's like walking on broken glass. Her skin can't be touched. It feels like a raw third-degree burn. Sleeping's impossible even with silk sheets. All she can do is scream. She'll lash out at anyone who talks to her. She's also angry at doctors because none of them has done anything for her."

It's not just Julie who needs therapy. Claudette talks without punctuation, her speech is jerky, and her voice trembles into a sound of love and frustration—a sign she's told her daughter's story too many times.

"Julie lost all her friends after the disease hit. She's trapped in pain while her friends go to college, vacation, or get jobs."

"How about online courses?"

"She registered for a couple, but she couldn't concentrate when the pain was so intense, which was almost daily."

Claudette gets misty-eyed when she recounts how she found Julie in the bathtub with her wrists slashed. "Thankfully, she was so dehydrated, the blood wouldn't run. She's still obsessed with death as her only escape."

I take advantage of the gap in her speech when she blows her nose. "How about your husband? How does he deal with it?"

"He pretends to work long hours and comes home after she's in bed. He can't handle seeing her suffer."

After Claudette leaves, I check my appearance in the mirror, color my lips pink, and ponder what to say to Julie before heading to her room. I knock at the door and a voice yells something unintelligible. Pushing the door open, I find Julie stretched on the bed playing a video game. She checks me out head to toe, then goes back to her screen.

"May I sit down?"

She rolls her eyes and jerks her head toward the chair. I sit down and talk with no plan. "What game are you playing?"

"Did my mother send you?"

"She did."

"I thought so. Can you give me a pair of legs?"

"No."

"Then get out. I don't need some psycho *merde*."

"I'm not here as your psychologist. I thought we could

talk as friends. I'm a patient, too."

"You can walk," she grunts.

"Not for long. You see..." I clear my throat to mask my tremulous voice. "I have a brain tumor that's probably getting bigger as we speak. There is a good chance I'll die in a few months."

"Then you're lucky." She adjusts her little body in the bed, throws the console on the pillow next to her, and turns to face me. "If you're dying, why are you here?"

"I can't let the disease win. I will fight until.... Dr. Hidalgo and Karina are very good at what they do. They treated people with all kinds of diseases who recovered. I believe I will beat cancer."

Julie ran out of words. Maybe I made a connection.

"Because everyone understands cancer! Nobody knows *CRPute*. I'm just some handicapped *merde* for the doctors to kick around."

"So, you think handicapped people are shit?"

"Dégages, connasse." She turns her head to the wall.

"Is that a compliment?" I grin. "I have a joke for you. Wanna hear it?"

"Comme tu veux," she whimpers, still staring at the wall.

"I'll take that as a yes. Here it goes. A man goes home and tells his wife: ' Honey, after three months of therapy, my therapist said something that brought tears to my eyes.' The wife looks at him with her eyes wide open. ' What did he say?'' *No hablo inglés*'."

Her eyes still on the tablet, Julie laughs, exposing her teeth for the first time.

"I have some good news for you. Your disease is caused by inflammation. From what I learned here, they can put it into remission."

She glares and grabs her console again. I continue talking while she tries to play her video game. "I took a lot of classes with Karina and Dr. Hidalgo and I learned about inflammation, antioxidants, and how food can heal you."

"Do you know how many charlatans we tried?" She lifts

her eyes from the console.

"Why did you accept to come here?"

"My mother said it's the last one. If it doesn't work, she'll help me die."

What words can I use to give her hope? Suddenly, something clicks in my head. Her despair is no different than mine. If I want to help Julie, I have to convince myself this treatment will work for me as well. Some days, I'm filled with hope, others, I'm hanging from a cliff. I leave Julie's room with more questions than answers.

I return to the computer and immerse myself in CRPS education. Scientific articles are scarce. The few sites that discuss the disease are from different hospitals such as the Mayo Clinic, Cleveland Clinic, and a few non-medical sites. The web pages mainly explain the symptoms and the different approaches to alleviate them. They all agree on one thing: there is no cure. I comb the web and scroll through the multitude of websites selling products, supplements, books, and even healing music.

I click on links until my fingers are sore. At the bottom of the twentieth page, a nutritionist website catches my eye. A sassy brunette with a large smile is the author of the article entitled *"Put CRPS in Remission."*

"CRPS is an inflammatory disease. An anti-inflammatory diet can soothe the pain, and for reasons unknown, the nerves can stop firing at random and resume normal functions. Scientific studies have established a correlation between pro-inflammatory foods and increased pain. Benefits of an anti-inflammatory diet include: prevention of further nerve damage, assistance in the healing of nerve damage...."

I review the scientific articles she linked and take copious notes.

The food this nutritionist promotes and the supplements she recommends are similar to what Dr. Hidalgo and Karina advise. I fold the sheet of paper and close the computer.

I walk to the dining room in search of Claudette. The patients are buzzing around, reading the ingredient lists and discussing the dishes. Everyone's present except Julie. Claudette stands in the back. I pull her aside and we sit on the other side of the pool.

"CRPS is an inflammatory disease caused by an injury to a nerve. "

"Julie developed the symptoms after a sprain. None of her doctors ever mentioned that it was inflammatory, much less discussing nutrition. They just kept prescribing meds."

"These are my notes about inflammation and how it can be tamed. Once the inflammation is under control, the nerves will eventually return to normal function. It's a slow process, but possible. Even if Julie doesn't take her supplements, just eating this food might improve her condition."

Claudette beams and breaks into tears. "I searched all over the internet and never found anything about nutrition. We've been passed around from doctor to doctor and everything I read on the web said it was hopeless."

"Nutrition is never included in medical treatment because dietitians have a very basic knowledge of nutrition and doctors don't respect them. Clinical nutritionists, like Karina, have a more advanced knowledge of the science of nutrition and understand how nutrients can reverse the course of a disease. What I've learned here is many conditions can be put into remission with just food."

"They wanted to remove the lymph nodes around her neck. That's the solution doctors came up with for the swelling."

"That would've been a huge mistake. Lymph node removal results in lymphedema. That's another nasty disease she doesn't need."

"What should I do now?" she asks after drying her tears.

"Have you talked to Dr. Hidalgo?"

"Not yet."

"He'll probably tell you to keep feeding her and let her vent. Once she feels a little better, she'll be motivated to comply. With Dr. Hidalgo's protocol, there is a good chance she'll walk again pain-free."

"I cannot thank you enough, Annie."

"You can. Teach me some French while you're here."

"Avec plaisir!"

We return to the lunch table. She immediately recognizes the Senegalese dishes. Her husband was a diplomat, and they lived in Senegal for several years and in the United States, which explains Julie's fluency in English.

Claudette smiles at how Chef Laora has reinvented traditional Senegalese cuisine. The famous chicken dish "poulet yassa" has become "tofu yassa"; the thiéboudieune—typically made of fresh and dried fish—is recreated with tempeh and seitan cooked with chayote fruit, cassava, and a variety of Andean potatoes served with a puree of garlic, onion, chilies, and tomato. A tureen holds another vegetable dish with peanut sauce called mafe topped with cilantro. The *pièce de résistance* is the dessert, captivating everyone's attention: a glass bowl with an orange rim filled with a creamy confection called clafoutis. It's made with almond and tapioca flours, hemp milk, and peaches. Oddly enough, it has a faint fragrance of eggs. After we devour the savory dishes, we race to the dessert bowl and make sure there isn't one morsel left.

ΛΛΛ

I open my eyes every morning to the warm rays of sunshine streaming through the round window. Ever since we connected, Daniel sends me a message, punctually at 7:00 a.m. before he goes to work. This morning, the clock says 7:00, but WhatsApp is mute. Probably an impromptu meeting or an unexpected event with Tanya. I linger in the room for an hour. Still nothing. I head out to breakfast. The room is deserted. I grab a couple of seed crackers and a banana and eat quickly by the pool. It's almost 9:00 and still no word from Daniel. In the entire time I've known him, he's never been late for anything, particularly with text messages. I mute the phone and walk to the yoga class.

I mechanically follow Diana's lead into each pose. I stretch my arms and legs into warrior one and two; we bend, monkey; we rise, mountain; face down for chaturanga, followed by cobra, up dog, down dog. I skip savasana and rush to check my phone. There is no orange number on the app. This is most unusual, so I send him a short message: *"Buenos dias, All OK with you*?" The message does not go through. A lonely check mark languishes on the screen. He must've turned off his phone. I shudder. No, his phone is always on.

Maybe he's just tired of me.

I replace lunch with a walk. I need to keep moving and help the clock along. I don't hear the birds tweeting and ignore the beautiful shy flowers spreading their little petals through the thin desert grass. I walk, check WhatsApp, and walk faster. Theories concerning his silence abound. What if he met someone vibrant and healthy? He's decided to end our relationship but doesn't know how to announce it. It's incompatible with his personality, but people's reactions are often out of character when they're uncomfortable.

Maybe something happened to Nina. Can't be. The last time we talked, he said she was better. I continue churning out theories and shutting them down. Then a crippling thought chills my blood. What if something happened to him? He could've been in an accident, incapacitated, or unable to communicate. I don't know anyone in his entourage.

Let's not panic. If I don't hear from him in a day or two, I'll locate his office and call them.

I walk the entire Paseo de la Serenidad, which ends in a plaza-like platform of beaten dirt strewn with pebbles and covered with a layer of orange dust, thinner than cake flour. A large, umbrella-like tree shelters it from the scorching sun. I crouch to rest in the shade. The Hill of Seven Colors stands in the distance. A large bird flies high in the sky, so close to the sun it could fry its wings. Complete tranquility, interrupted only by insects running under the brush. Using a twig, I draw shapes in the powdery dust. I trace long lines, short lines, and circles and join them to create some abstract geometry. I'm startled by WhatsApp's joyful chirp. I open the app and there he is. I breathe deep and swallow to moisten my dust-covered throat before reading the message.

Sorry, cara. In ER most of night. Nina passed away early this morning. I'll b n touch soon.

He logs off before I have a chance to reply.

My brain hits pause. I stare at the phone screen, weightless, immobilized, like a dry autumn leaf hardened by the frost. I sink deeper into the orange powder without feeling the pebbles digging into my skin. When I breathe again, I sob loudly, abundantly. I cry for Nina and for the life she'll never have; I cry for me and the future I lost; I cry longer; I cry more. A breeze sweeps my face. My hands turned orange and powdery. I dry my face with my forearms.

I sober up and slowly rise to walk back to my room, hoping not to run into anyone. After a shower, I stretch on the bed and spend the rest of the afternoon alone watching Hitchcock's *Rebecca*.

/\ /\ /\

It's been three days since Nina passed away. Three long days without hearing from him. I keep busy by attending all the offered activities; reading is a challenge due to my brain wandering off. I check WhatsApp almost every minute. My last message has still not been received. Without access to any information, my mind becomes prolific with theories to scare myself. What if he feels guilty about our relationship? Maybe he wants to be single for a while. Nina may occupy more space in his life now than when she was alive. I want to be prepared for whatever decision he makes.

I walk to Julie's room to check on her. I had another meeting with Claudette yesterday. Julie has been eating everything brought to her and even ventured out for a meal.

I knock at her door and Julie answers with a calm voice.

"Oui?"

"How are you, Julie?"

She's sitting on the covers with her knees up and her feet flat on the bed. She mumbles, "Alive."

"You can put your feet down now?"

"Only on the bed. It still hurts if I step on the floor."

I have a plan: get her to talk about her feelings toward the disease, help her visualize it, and guide her toward a more positive thought pattern. But first, I need to establish trust.

"So, do you have a boyfriend?" she asks, making eye contact for the first time.

"How is that relevant?" I reply, baffled.

"You said you wanted to be my friend."

"Fair enough. I do see someone. But there is nothing he can do about cancer. Having a boyfriend is not always a key to happiness; sometimes, it's the opposite."

"He's not good in bed, huh!" She smirks as she turns her head to face me.

"I don't know. What's your criteria?"

Julie giggles and blushes. "I never dated. Well, once when I was seventeen, but we didn't even kiss. Then I got sick. Now, I don't even have a friend."

"There are many people who are in wheelchairs, who have their arms amputated or disfigured by fire, and they still manage to find love and build a circle of friends."

"Right, all I have to do is be nice!" She raises her arms to the sky.

"Not a bad place to start. Everyone here is sick, Julie, and some of us will not recover."

She pauses. I seize the opportunity to lead her away from the anger. "So, let's dial time forward to when you're no longer sick. What would you like to accomplish? Where would you go on vacation?"

Projecting herself in a healthy state puts Julie in a better mood. Her jaw loosens and her brown eyes brighten. She talks with softer lips and a lower voice. "I want to go to the beach and walk barefoot on the sand. I would love to take a shower and feel water running on my skin. Haven't done that in years."

She's still skeptical about nutrition therapy until I remind her she's not living up to the agreement she made with her mother.

"If you don't adhere to the program and participate, your mother doesn't have to keep her word."

"Fine! I'll talk to the doctor tomorrow."

"Karina is here. You can talk to her today and get some supplements right away."

ΛΛΛ

After lunch, Donna and I sit by the pool sipping Chef Laora's special cocktails: fizzy water, cucumber, and mint, infused with passion fruit extract. We both agree it needs more sugar and vodka. Donna scans me head to toe before initiating her investigative questioning. "You disappeared yesterday. Is everything OK?"

"I've not heard from Daniel in a couple of days. Some family problems..."

She lifts her chin. "Married or divorced?"

"Widowed."

"Honey, those are the best. They can commit and the wife didn't take any of the assets."

"Isn't that macabre?"

"There's always a silver lining. You just have to find it."

Donna speaks her mind with the honesty of a child. She may sound judgmental at times, but beneath the rough exterior, she's a marshmallow. Discussing Julie and Claudette's turmoil, she gets misty-eyed. She recalls how her illness affected her daughter, who was only thirteen when the fatigue started.

"Annie, you've been counseling everyone since you've been here. Who's counseling you?"

"My work is my therapy."

ΛΛΛ

Day five without any news from Daniel. My anxiety has reached its peak. It's now stable. I run out of theories and just check WhatsApp regularly. In an act of desperation to kill time faster, I attend the morning meditation class. Sitting in a quiet room with my eyes closed and trying to clear my mind of chatter is a challenge, but I have exhausted all other avenues. Besides, this is exactly what meditation should do: relieve anxiety and open the path for rational and purposeful thinking.

I sit in the back so only Diana can see me. With our legs folded into a lotus position and our eyes closed, we listen to Diana's voice guiding us to breathe, clear our minds, and feel grounded.

I sit with my eyes downcast, tears streaming and collecting on my neck. Then Diana looks at me and points a finger to the door behind me. Camila, the new hire who doesn't speak English, motions for me to follow her.

My negative energy sent vibes through the room. I should be removed to not contaminate others.

I tiptoe out and follow Camila. She's saying something in Spanish with a smile that illuminates her beautiful face. I walk behind her, through the hallway, to the reception office. She opens the door and leads me out.

I float out of my body and look down. He's standing in front of a rental car—meditation worked, after all. Feet glued to the ground, I use my hand to shield my eyes from the sunlight. He walks toward me. We hug strongly—intensely. There is no noise, no wind, only the birds singing. The warmth of the sun wraps us in soft colors. Words are unnecessary—none would fit the circumstances. I pull away to look at his face, but he just stares at his shoes. He then lifts his head to say something, but I put my hand on his lips.

"You're here now. That's all I need to know."

He takes my hand and leads us to the car.

"How's Tanya?" I ask as soon as the doors close.

"It was expected, but it's still rough on her. She's only sixteen."

I put my head on his shoulder and we sit there in silence. Then he pulls away, which always makes me feel rejected. During his previous visits, at every departure, I sat next to him in the car and locked his arm between mine to hold on to him a little longer. To signal his readiness to leave, he would wiggle out his arm and turn on the ignition. I felt pushed away.

"You have ten minutes to get dressed for the desert and grab your sunglasses. I am kidnapping you for the day."

"I don't think I'm allowed to leave."

"It's taken care of."

He goes to the reception desk to sign forms and I run back to my room and change into hiking gear: jeans, sneakers, hair styled in a ponytail, face dressed with sunscreen, lipstick, and sunglasses. I return to the car and throw my purse in the back seat. Before he cranks the engine, I say, "I can't believe you're here! Where are you taking me?"

He kisses my forehead and starts the car. "To Serrania del Hornocal. Also known as the Hill of Fourteen Colors. It's five thousand meters above sea level. I think it translates to something like sixteen thousand feet."

We drive north of Jujuy. The sun is shining so brightly, the only sign of yesterday's rain are puddles and mud on the road. A little frown draws his eyebrows closer. His face sags a little and has a gray tone, like someone who has not slept for days. He's quieter than usual, more focused, and withdrawn. He lets me hold his hand without a response—no squeeze, no kiss, no movement.

As a psychologist, I understand the stages of grief he's going through; as his girlfriend, I resent he's grieving the loss of another woman. Human feelings are complex and often shamefully ugly.

This impromptu visit is probably a goodbye date. He has too much class to break up over the phone or on video. Why would he want to be with someone of reduced life expectancy again when he can have any woman he wants? I prepare myself for the long breakup speech. I let go of his hand and pull away to the corner of the car between the seat and the door. He doesn't notice. If he's dumping me with class, I have to respond in kind. My only problem is how to get back to the center. I don't want to drive back with him after he "discards" me.

I turn my head to the window to immerse myself in the surrounding landscape. We take Route 9 north through neighborhoods lined with adobe homes pierced with low windows and vibrantly painted doors at street level. Most buildings are white with bleeding orange streaks formed by water dragging dust down the walls, giving them an orange-brownish base. A few homes have a cement structure, no paint, all gray with a stone base.

We reach the ancient town of Tilcara. The road is bordered by small buildings—homes and stores—sprinkled with tall trees adorned with wispy leaves. In the distance, a panoramic view of the Serrania del Hornocal opens up. It's a spectacle of colors with triangles neatly stacked against each other, forming a canvas of warm hues ranging from orange to purple to grayish blue. We drive in silence through narrow streets and pass people carrying shopping bags, women with toddlers strapped to their backs, and herd animals grazing freely. He slows down to avoid bumping into them. The greenery contrasts with the rugged surrounding hills with bold tops. The rainbow-colored rock formations, the unspoiled landscape, and the indigenous architecture make driving through this ancient town a National Geographic experience.

His eyes focused on the road, he gives me the background history. "This is called the Quebrada de Humahuaca. It's now declared a UNESCO World Heritage. It's one of the rare places in the world that preserves the ancient indigenous culture. The town of Tilcara has experienced continuous inhabitation that can be traced back ten thousand years."

I feel queasy; I ask him to slow down.

He hands me a bag of candy. "Try one of these. It helps with the altitude."

We arrive at an outdoor market. Another moment worth framing in a travel magazine. Chickens running everywhere; children wearing T-shirts with inscribed American cities: New York City, Los Angeles, Miami. Women cooking on hot plates or open fire. Appetizing chicken skewers, empanadas, eggs, and various dishes generously spread their aroma to entice the hungry traveler.

I ask, "Can we stop and browse?"

He smiles. "I promised I'd keep you safe. No interaction with people. Just you and me."

When Daniel gives his word, it's a binding contract.

We ascend a hill and he squirts water on the windshield to wash away the cocoa-like powder. It makes a paste that smears all over the windshield. More water dilutes it into orange streams the wipers sweep to the side.

About forty-five minutes on the road, past Tilcara and the small adobe village of Huacalera, he opens up a little.

"Tanya is having a difficult time coping. She's been glued to me for the last three days. She has even slept with me for two nights."

"Where's she now?"

"Her grandparents insisted on taking her for a few days."

"How are the in-laws"?

"Same as usual. They blame me for the accident, and now they're angry because I respected her wishes to be cremated."

"I suppose you didn't have a funeral."

He slouches back in his seat. "Group gatherings are still not allowed. So, I spent the last few days answering calls and emails from people who wanted to send flowers or make donations."

"She must've been very popular."

"She was the type of person everyone wanted as a friend,

always happy, generous, and never complained about anything. She used to say ' *no hay problema, solo hay soluciones* —' there are no problems, only solutions."

I'm not sure why he needs to fill me in on the type of person she was, but I asked. I received. The heat and the dust dry my mouth. I extend my hand to reach for a bottle of water in the backseat.

"See? That's why I didn't contact you the last few days." He sighs in a reprimanding tone, assuming I am upset.

"Honey, I don't mind you talking about Nina. You shared a life with her... and a child."

He ignores me and stares at the wheel. The only noise that cuts the thick silence is the crunching of pebbles and twigs under the tires.

We cross another little town, Humahuaca, to drive east on Route 73, which leads to the viewing platform. Clouds of dust rise and cover the windows. Driving through unpaved pebbly switchbacks makes me dizzy. I hold onto the seat and distract myself by looking through the almost opaque windows at the cacti with their beautiful red fruit, llamas grazing in the distance, and the vibrant red peaks barely visible through the haze. He occasionally asks how I'm feeling, but there is no warmth in his voice. Despite the bumpy ride, my mental discomfort is greater than my physical one.

After what seems like hours of slow driving, we arrive at the park entrance, where we pay a fee to enter. When we finally reach the top of the mountain, I'm out of breath, both literally and figuratively. Then I'm face to face with the majestic mountain. It displays way over fourteen colors, possibly twenty or more. The triangles line up neatly into a zig-zag pattern from one side to the other, making a stark contrast to the green tapestry of grass with rough bristles. He reaches to hold my hand and I just stand still, immobilized, in awe of nature's masterpiece.

"Are you okay?" he asks.

"Just overwhelmed. Never seen anything like it."

"There is an even better view about three hundred meters down, but it's a very steep slope."

We walk away to avoid the small group of tourists chatting and taking pictures. He's brought a blanket, which we put on the short, thin grass. He also has a hat for me and bottles of water. As soon as we sit down, he begins what I expected.

"I wanted to spend the day with you because—"

"It's okay, there's no need to explain. I'm prepared to let you go," I reply in a cold, stern voice as I lift my eyes toward the crown of the hill and swallow the lump in my throat. How I wish I was like my mother!

He's taken aback. His whole face wrinkles as he squints in an inquisitive glare. "Let me go where?"

"Set you free so you can find happiness with someone healthier."

"Dios! You thought I brought you here to break us up?"

This is the first time I see him angry. Not sure what to do, I grab a bottle of water and gulp it down.

He shakes his head and rubs his temples in exasperation. "What I wanted to tell you, is I won't be able to come see you for the remainder of your stay here. I have to take care of Tanya, find her counseling, and take her out of Buenos Aires on weekends."

I rise to my knees to face him and throw my arms around his neck to hold tight. Then I offer my explanation, which infuriates him even more. "You were so quiet in the car, so I thought..."

"I woke up at 4:00 a.m.! I was trying to keep my eyes open on the road!" he roars. "Why can't you accept the fact that I love you?"

"I may not make it and I don't want you to go through this again."

"I don't regret one minute I spent with Nina in the last ten years. It's not the life we planned, but love is not a market where you take back what didn't fit."

"You have to see this from my end. You disappear for

days, then you show up completely shut down."

"I'm sorry. I didn't think of how it would affect you. I wanted to shield you from the whole madness. It was sad and busy; the house was full of people all the time; Tanya was inconsolable; I've gotten maybe eight hours of sleep in the last four days."

"I guess you're right. I only think about myself."

He smiles and puts his hand on my neck. "No, you're right, I should've contacted you. Please forgive me."

"I will, but it'll cost you."

Our conversation pattern is restored and we're back to our old emotional space. But he's grieving and clearly feels awkward sharing his sorrow with me.

"Honey, I don't need to be sheltered. I know how close you and your wife were. She was a great mother, your best friend, and sounds like an exceptional person in many ways."

"She was all that and more, and that's all I'll say about it."

His eyes fill with tears, but he keeps looking straight into my eyes. I wipe away the tears, kiss his lips softly, then put my head on his knees with my arms wrapped around them.

A bout of fatigue creeps up. The emotional roller coaster and the altitude have depleted my low energy reserves. I have some big shoes to fill, but I can shrink them.

8 - Microriche for All

We leave the magical mountains and head down to the little town of Humahuaca for lunch. A drive that should last ten minutes takes almost an hour on the winding, unpaved roads. Trucks and tourist buses come straight at us; when they're within a few inches from our windshield, they swerve and almost brush against our car. Skilled Argentinian drivers leave only millimeters between themselves and other vehicles. Daniel smiles when I cover my eyes.

In Humahuaca, more dirt roads outline orange and pink adobe buildings, with Spanish churches rising in the distance. We reach a small cluster of homes and, after a few turns, we arrive at the back of a hamlet. He parks in front of a small rambler with short lime-painted walls and small windows barely off the ground. We follow a narrow dirt path to a pink door behind a tall tree surrounded by blooming plants and desert brush. Daniel twists the doorknob and motions for me to enter.

"Don't they lock their doors?" I ask as I step on the cement floor.

"The owner is my friend Diego's aunt. She left the door unlocked for us. She's staying with her sister two houses down. All the neighbors are related in one way or another. Burglary is extremely rare around here."

"You have nice friends."

"Diego stayed three months in my house during his divorce."

We step directly into a small kitchen with a gas stove and shelves holding the kitchen utensils—no cabinets. Scarves and ponchos hang on pegs along the back wall. A door to the left of the kitchen opens on the bedrooms and bathroom.

Diego's aunt prepared lunch for us ahead of time. She also set the table for us: pottery plates, bowls, a basket of fruit, platters of tamales, and empanadas covered with Andean-style napkins.

Daniel moves to the stove, lifts the lid, looks inside, then replaces it. "Locro. Good, she made it vegan."

"What is locro?"

"A traditional stew. It's usually made with pork, chorizo, chickpeas, lima beans, and hominy. It's a hearty cold-weather dish, but the vegan version is lighter." He turns on the stove to warm the stew while I fill the glasses with water.

The delicious aroma from the pot stokes my appetite. Diego's aunt is a talented cook. She converted traditional meals into vegan ones and made them just as delicious. The locro is creamy with chunks that resemble kabocha squash and the lima beans are still chewy. The tamales are a novelty to me. Made with cornmeal and spices and steamed in a corn husk, they delicately melt in the mouth.

After we sample everything, he asks, "How old were you when your parents adopted you?"

"A couple of weeks. Why?"

"Have you ever thought about finding your birth parents?"

"Where is this coming from?"

"You have fear of abandonment."

"I do not!"

"Annie?" He bowed his head to give me a skeptical glare. "You know I'm right."

"I grew up with the best parents a child could ever want."

He caresses my cheek and smiles. "I'm here to stay—until you tire of me."

He sees through my insecurities but reached the wrong assumption. The reality is, I've never been this deeply in love, and with a man grieving a superwoman. Then there is my defective health. When I do the math, I have little to offer. "Well, you're the only Argentinian I know. How can I be sure you're even a good Argentinian?"

"I assure you, I'm the best the country can produce."

"Bueno! In that case, I'll keep you."

It suddenly dawns on me that he went through so much trouble to organize a day for us that still keeps me isolated. I've been so wrapped up in my fears, I haven't even acknowledged his efforts.

"This is an amazing day. You really put a lot of work into it."

"It's tough being at Años Mejores without visitors. I wanted to at least get you out for one day."

"The first couple of weeks were rough, but I've gotten used to it now. It's been almost two months. It's not so bad."

"You're about to lose me," he says, lifting his eyebrows to prevent the eyelids from covering the eyes.

I help him stand up and guide him toward the bedroom. "Okay, old man, lean on my shoulder."

As soon as his head reaches the pillow, he falls asleep before he's fully horizontal. I remove his shoes and watch him sink into a deep sleep.

I clear the table and cover the remaining food. Outside, I take pictures of the house and the surroundings, the hills, the quaint houses, and the streets. I'm not much into social media posting, but I want to frame the moment and share all the unique beauty of the Andean landscape with the world. Twenty minutes later, my pictures received dozens of likes and over thirty comments from people telling me to enjoy my vacation. Social media is like an aerial view of life: only the big picture is visible.

A crowing rooster wakes Daniel an hour later. This bird's call signals the end of the afternoon. I enter the bedroom and find him rubbing his eyes to shake off the last remnants of sleep. I lie next to him and we kiss. We hold each other tight to find our closeness again. I want to stretch this moment, but as usual, we have to race against the clock. He pulls away from me, puts his shoes on, and we drive back to my cell.

/\ /\ /\

We arrive at Años Mejores just before sunset. I hold on to him for a few more minutes, knowing that delaying his departure could result in a missed flight. Then I exit the car and watch him drive away. Suddenly, I have an urge to tell him how much I love him. I run after the car. He stops and rolls down the window.

"I lied. I can't let you go. I never thought I'd love anyone this much."

He extends his arm to caress my face. He purses his lips and nods in agreement. "Give me time to sort through all this."

"You got it."

"We can still Zoom and talk on the phone, okay?"

"Por supuesto…" I watch the car disappear in an orange cloud, and my heart feels big again.

A small card is attached to my door: an invitation to celebrate Ernesto's departure. As much as I'm happy for him, I've grown attached to the old man. He's everyone's friend. He always has something nice to say, a joke, a compliment. AM will be boring without him.

ΛΛΛ

We gather at the swimming pool. Stefani and Sonia have put balloons and flowers around the table with a giant three-layer coconut-passion fruit cake in the center. A terra cotta cazuela dish—a Spanish hybrid of plate and bowl with a handle on each side—holds a coconut-cream sauce topping.

Donna arrives, and for the first time, she's wearing black pants and a red tank top. She greets me with her usual bright smile as she twirls in front of me.

"I lost twenty pounds. Can you believe it?"

"You look stunning!"

"I never thought it would happen. Dr. Hidalgo says my metabolism is now fired up and the weight will continue to drop and my energy will keep climbing."

"How's the pain?"

"Non existent. No more joint pain, no more bloat-ing—well, I still have this hanging belly, but all the bloating is gone. It's mostly fat now. I can walk, swim, and stand for hours. When I came here, I used a wheelchair at the airport. I couldn't stand in line."

Both staff and patients have come to wish Ernesto well. Dr. Hidalgo moves toward us. He's wearing black trousers and an ironed and starched purple shirt. His wavy hair is longer and covers his neck and ears. He compliments Donna on her beautiful complexion and weight loss. Her eyes are livelier, and even her posture is better.

"Do you take before and after pictures?" I ask.

"These things can't be captured by a camera. You see, when people have inflammation, their tone is gray, their eyeballs are yellow, their smile is tired, and the texture of the skin is spongy or dull. Not something you can see in pictures."

He smiles at me. "How are you, Annie?" His voice shivers a little.

"I feel much better. I sleep more soundly and have more energy every day," I reply before Karina cuts in to congratulate me on my progress. Then Sylvia joins us. She and I have not interacted much. She's also radiant and is probably about to leave as well. A tap on my shoulder startles me and I almost scream as I turn. Julie stands without crutches.

"I can walk, Annie."

She has lost the hardened shell that covered her personality. Her smile is warm, and her eyes are open wider and brighter.

"You have legs!"

"First time in years. It still hurts, but I can stand and walk for a few minutes."

"I think she's on her way now. She's definitely more motivated," Claudette says, her voice warm and hopeful. "I don't know what you told her, but she's more positive than I've seen her in years."

"I just allowed her to vent."

Once everyone has arrived, Diana brings Ernesto, whom she kept occupied by pretending she needed help to move boxes. Ernesto never turns away anyone needing help. As soon as we see him, we all scream "Felicidades!" He's visibly emotional when he sees the festive atmosphere.

Chef Laora distributes plates with cake slices and we add our own sauce. Pablo is first in line; he tops his cake with coconut sauce and, as always, sits alone. Donna and I walk to the other side of the pool to enjoy the long chairs. When I mention Pablo to Donna, she almost scolds me.

"Whatever you do," she orders, "don't talk to Picasso."

"Why not?"

"I don't want him to get you all depressed. He has jaw cancer." She sighs. "They removed the bone in his left jaw and replaced it with a piece of bone from his leg. They told him if the cancer came back, they'd remove half his face. So, his wife freaked out and left him. He's constantly moping about her. Pathetic."

"You can miss someone who doesn't love you."

"Sorry. Don't get that. If someone leaves you when you're sick, you've been with the wrong person all along. Control Alt Delete."

"Sorry, I have a Mac."

"Even better: killall."

"Translation, Silicon Valley girl!"

"It's a Unix command that terminates all running processes."

We continue to dig through the layers of the cake and delight in the sweetness of the moment. Suddenly, Donna jumps to her feet.

"It's a beautiful evening. Let's walk. I'm like a toddler who just discovered the power of her little legs. I want to walk every day."

We walk the Paseo de la Serenidad. Both the sun and the heat have abated, leaving a translucent orange light almost like candlelight. The tranquility is both romantic and haunting—a reminder of loneliness.

Donna sniffs the desert air. "I'm craving chicken."

"You need help for those dark thoughts."

"It'd better come in a bucket of fried chicken. I'm going to ask John Henry over there." She points back toward the compound.

"Who's John Henry?"

"The gardener. I call him John Henry the Steel Man because he's all muscles and he likes to show them off. He wears those tank tops with very thin straps to show his biceps and pecs."

"I think it's because he's hot."

"I *think* I can bribe him into buying me some chicken."

"Donna? That's breaking the rules."

"Oh, hush, Janet."

"Janet? Is that my nickname now?"

"Yeah, you're tall and always proper, obeying all the rules."

"You know chicken has arachidonic acid. You will be shamed and probably tortured for such transgression."

"I can see Karina with her whip all dressed in kale."

"The whip is certified plant-based."

"I know, organic poison ivy."

We laugh loudly until the mountain echoes our voices.

"You don't have a common language. How will you ask him to buy you anything?"

"Dineros and Google translator."

"I think they're called pesos here. He could lose his job, you know."

"I'm in Argentina, damn it! Best meat in the world. I'll get me some."

We keep walking. She stops and picks a small flower from the bushes and puts it behind her ear. Then turns toward me.

"I need to talk to you about something."

"You're craving bacon now?"

"Remember how I told you I wanted to start a business? Well, it came to me two nights ago. I want to create a non-profit organization devoted to patient education. I also want clinics staffed with nutritionists, functional medicine doctors, and chefs to transition people to healthy eating."

"That's a huge endeavor that'll require a lot of funds."

"I know pretty much everyone in Silicon Valley. I'm not as hot as Elizabeth Holmes, but I can sell ice to Eskimos, sand to the Bedouins."

"Yeah, but could you sell a PC to Steve Jobs?"

"I could sell him an iPC!" Donna pauses, then pushes her hair back, lifts her chin, and opens her eyes wide as if she just remembered something important. "You know who could help with that? Melinda."

"Melinda Gates?"

"Yeah. She's all about health. We used to work together."

"Are you close friends?"

She shrugged. "We stayed in touch over the years."

"And I can draft in Barack Obama. He's my neighbor, ya know!" While I'm joking, Donna thinks it's not a bad idea to contact Michelle Obama—another woman concerned with the environment and healthy eating.

We arrive at the Plaza and sit on the new bench beneath the tree. Donna is ignited. She lays out the business plan, people she can reach out to for funding, people she can hire, the size of the clinics, and training for the staff. We sit on the bench for about an hour and Donna talks in one breath.

"Annie, there is a part in this for you, too. I want you to join me as a co-founder."

"I'm a psychologist. I know nothing about business."

"You're a doctor. You can develop training material for the staff, lecture series, and help recruit a board of directors. Most importantly, you'll help put together a team of clinicians. I'll manage everything on thc business side, and you'll manage the clinical side of the operation."

"It does sound tempting."

"You see, people scream socialized medicine anytime someone wants to make a change to our archaic, obsolete, abusive medical system and that's bull. We have primitive medicine in the US. Doctors are mechanics with narrow tunnel vision. When you present them with a problem not on their tiny list, if they can't hand you a pill, they'll discard you like garbage."

"That hasn't been my experience."

"You're young and beautiful. You also have something they understand. Try talking to them about swelling, pain, screwed up digestion, or something unexplained. If you're my age and overweight, they'll blame you for being fat and dismiss your complaints as menopause. D'you know how aggravating that is? When you're suffering every day and you're told it's because you're old and fat?"

"Doctors don't like to feel powerless."

"Right! So, they blame the patient for their impotence. My friend Lisa had a swollen foot; then, the entire leg became swollen. Her doctor told her it was just cosmetic and she could live with it. She's seen five doctors. None of them gave her a diagnosis. She spent a fortune on all kinds of charlatans who promised to balance her energy and clean her chakras. She even bought some kind of water that was supposed to improve her cellular health. She eventually went to see a podiatrist because she developed infections in her foot that festered. He diagnosed her with lymphedema."

As she moves through the story, her voice rises, profanities fly out, and her anger culminates into a frightening hate. This funny and sarcastic woman becomes a powerful fireball that could set this dry land ablaze.

"I agree. Sometimes they miss things."

"Tell me about it. The podiatrist told her if it had been treated when it first appeared, it would've been controlled. The disease has now advanced and the skin has become thick and hard or something; she's in constant pain and getting more infections."

"She developed fibrosis. How is she now?"

"Last time I talked to her, she was going to attempt surgery. All this could've been prevented if the motherfuckers did their job!"

"I'm so sorry about your friend."

"Don't be sorry. Let's do something. Millions of people

suffer every day, putting their trust in the hands of incompetent robots. You and I are rich and educated, and we know how to sift through information and find the right help."

"Rich? Excuse me?"

"Honey, if you can afford to take three months off and drop eight grand on this place, you're rich. Most people can't afford rent and they're struggling with the same shit we are. They don't have time to browse the internet and, when they do, they have no idea what's true and what's bullshit. It took me a year to find this place. Then I read reviews, bios, and asked other professionals. Most people don't have the bandwidth for such scrutiny. Out of desperation, they'll attempt anything to get relief. They eventually fall victim to crooks."

"Believe me, I know. So many of my patients tell me about a new tea, some powder from an exotic plant they found online, or some supplement because there is no medication for what they have."

"I want a place that will do this type of research for people. Identify their ailment and investigate all possible solutions, risks, and benefits. I want to counsel cancer patients before treatment so they're aware of all the side effects and what changes to expect down the road. If Lisa was warned about the effects of radiation, she would've taken precautions to prevent the disease or refuse treatment."

"The treatment saved her life, though."

"She should've been informed of the risks. If she was prepared, she could've prevented the disease from progressing. Her leg started swelling twelve years after the cancer treatment." Donna shakes her head and sighs. "Please say you'll do this with me."

An electric current runs down my spine whenever someone talks about the future. The amount of time I have left could be counted in months on fingers. I hold on to hope like a drawing woman holds on to a splintering branch.

"Donna, I don't know—"

"You'll make it. It has worked for everyone else. Please don't say no."

"Fine, I'm in. Tentatively. I do have a lot of questions, though. Another reason I hesitate—"

"You're not getting married, are you?"

I laugh. "No. I'm worried about my health."

My entire body twitches at the idea of marrying Daniel. We've never discussed the future, but like a subconscious image or an earlier life memory, it does drop in my mind from time to time like a flying spark from burning wood.

I ask, "Do I have to move to California?"

"Not initially. You can work remotely until we have the funds to pay you a salary. Then you'll have to move to wherever we set up the office and our pilot clinic."

"Can you move to Virginia?"

"Most of my contacts are in California—a few in New York."

Once I gear the conversation toward business, Donna regains her cheerful attitude. We continue chewing on ideas until I lift my eyes to the sky.

"Donna, look!"

A ball of fire illuminates the sky and an impressionist canvas emerges with dozens of shades of orange, purple, soft blue, and red. We stare at it, mesmerized and our hearts filled with hope.

ΛΛΛ

Karina has a powerful blender on the working station to prepare for the ice cream class. Sylvia sits in the front row, eager to absorb every bit of Karina's wisdom. Most shocking of all is Julie's attendance. Donna rolls her eyes at the display of fruit and nut milks.

"I'm actually excited to learn about making non-dairy ice cream. I always feel bloated after eating ice cream. My belly has been completely flat since I've been here."

"I'll keep an open mind, but nothing can replace real

French vanilla ice cream," Donna says. "My previous doctors told me I had IBS, but Dr. Hidalgo said all the symptoms would disappear once I stopped eating dairy."

As much as Donna and I want to deny it, we don't miss meat or cheese. Our taste buds have changed and adapted to different flavors. Contrary to what one would think, the food tastes better. With so many colorful dishes and flavors to explore, it's never boring or monotonous.

Karina begins with everyone's favorite: chocolate ice cream. Chocolate has antioxidants and minerals and is therapeutic. It's not always a dessert. Without the addition of sugar and milk, it can be added to savory dishes and pairs well with beans, rice, chili peppers, corn, and fruit such as pears and strawberries. Unlike the smooth, velvety texture we're accustomed to, when raw and pure, chocolate is grainy and has a slight sandy texture.

She pours cashew milk and ice cubes into the blender and adds vanilla extract, cocoa nibs, a couple of dates, and cocoa powder. She runs the blender until all the ingredients form one homogenous concoction. Sonia scoops the ice cream into ramekins and passes them out.

The creamy chocolate melts in the mouth into layers of deep chocolate, vanilla, and rum, and finishes with a light caramel. The bitterness of the chocolate is perfectly balanced with the sweetness of the dates and vanilla, unlike traditional ice cream, which often has a sugar aftertaste without any variation.

Donna raises her eyebrows with surprise and approval and joins me for seconds.

After the chocolate comes strawberry and coconut ice cream, acai sorbet, and the all-so-familiar vanilla ice cream topped with Goji berry marmalade. She finishes the class with a word of caution: even though these ice cream recipes are healthful, they still have a good amount of sugar, and indulging in them regularly will not lead to disease, but can increase our weight.

After the class, Donna invites me to her room, claiming

she has a surprise for me.

"Wait till you see this," she says as she reaches under the bed. She draws out a small box, which she opens wide.

"Fried chicken, baby!"

My stomach turns and acid rises into my esophagus. Hand to mouth, I run to the bathroom. I gag and nearly vomit, but thankfully nothing comes up.

I wipe my lips as I emerge from the bathroom. "I'm sorry. I can no longer tolerate the smell of chicken."

"You're pregnant," she crows with a loud laugh and collapses on the bed. "Honey, you're having a baby."

"No, there's no baby."

"Are you sure?"

"Yes, as of three days ago."

"Oh. Then you've been a vegan in the closet all your life?" She pauses and twists her mouth into a grimace. "Well, tell you the truth, it's not as good as I expected." She shakes the small glistening pieces in the box, closes it, and puts it in the trash bin.

"What d'you know! We're vegan."

"I don't feel as stuffy after eating anymore. I don't think I'll go back to eating animal foods and, if the tumor in my brain shrinks, that's a bonus."

"OK, let's talk business."

She opens a PowerPoint presentation of her business plan and describes the steps involved in putting together a new association. Talking about business is usually boring, but with Donna, it's poetry.

"Here's the executive summary."

"Just one paragraph?"

"This is like an elevator speech. It's the first thing we tell potential sponsors, members, and anyone we need support from. It's a short description of our services."

Without catching a breath, she scrolls down to pages and pages of graphs, pictures, and tables. "I've also done market analysis. There is nothing like this out there."

"How about the American Heart Association, the American Diabetes Association, the Lupus Foundation?"

"There are all kinds of foundations, but all they do is raise money to finance the foundation. None of them provide patient services and each foundation addresses one specific health problem. If doctors don't give you a diagnosis, where do you go?"

"I think their purpose is to raise awareness and fund research projects. The information is educational. It's not intended to treat."

"Exactly. Fuck that. A lot of those organizations are corrupt and the funds go to pay salaries of top executives. They spend all their time on fundraising rather than providing useful information to patients. We're creating a space for patients to discuss all their conditions with a knowledgeable health practitioner who can guide them in their treatment program. We'll put in place a Patient Care Adviser who will interview the patient, record all the symptoms, and all the changes since the problem occurred, collect demographics, and perform an assessment. Then she will make recommendations on which healthcare provider the patient needs to contact for a confirmed diagnosis, tests, and treatment. We'll have a list of practitioners from all kinds of professions: therapists, doctors, surgeons, nutritionists."

"How about liability?"

"We won't provide any diagnosis or treatment. Our lawyer will draft a disclaimer and whatever we need to protect ourselves. Our job is to provide the patient with answers and guidance about the right treatment for them and where to get it. Then put them in touch with the appropriate provider. If someone calls with strange symptoms and her doctor is telling her nothing can be done, we will dig until we find a solution for that person. Then we will match them with a health care provider specialized in that disease."

"Can we add a shaman to the list?" I giggle. "I always wanted to consult a shaman."

"I'm serious, Annie. We can build an organization that

can serve as the first point of contact for all these people with weird health problems that conventional medicine can't treat. You see, if someone told poor Claudette where to go, her daughter could've been helped years ago."

"So, you want to identify the exact health problem and connect people with the right health professional."

"Exactly. No more guessing, no more scrolling through pages and pages of bullshit on the internet. We will have educated and trained people to do all that legwork and find the information the patient needs along with all the treatment options available to them before referring them to the corresponding health professional."

"Kinda like a 911 for health."

Donna beams. "Hmm. You know, that could be a good URL, too. 911YourHealth.com"

She has identified a niche where the association can thrive; she's already drafted a list of people to contact for funding and created a step-by-step plan on how to market the association.

"The second part of the association will be devoted to teaching people how to modify their diet and eat healthy. We'll need chefs, nutritionists, and functional medicine doctors specialized in the Microriche diet."

When she opens the finance spreadsheet, she sees my enthusiasm waning.

"Donna, I love the idea, but I'll leave the finances to you."

"Fair enough."

She closes the laptop and, with a radiant smile, proclaims, "We're partners. When we get home, I'll have a lawyer draft a contract to send to you."

"I'll sign after I see the MRI results."

"You'll be fine. Don't worry so much." She reopens the laptop. "I forgot. We have to find a name for the association."

We brainstorm for over two hours and veto every name we come up with. Then we make a list of words and arrange them in a different order to form acronyms composed of all the words we want in the title, something easy for people to remember and short to put in a URL. Our word list includes *healing, pain, medical, patients, network, organization, advocacy, health, people*.

"People's Advocacy Network. Neh, scratch that. Apostrophes make a name heavy and awkward. How about patient health… something? I want the word patient there. I'm thinking…" Then Donna zeroes in on three words: Patient Education Network: PEN.

"Love it. Simple and easy to remember."

"It's perfect for a URL. With long names, people make mistakes when typing them into the browser. On the other hand, the acronym doesn't say what we do. It's a bit banal. Let's type that into whois."

"Whois who is? Sorry, I couldn't resist."

"It's a site where you check if a domain name is available."

It's mesmerizing to watch Donna at work. She has a plethora of ideas and can argue the pros and cons of each; she explains her reasoning behind each word, how it will play a role in search engine optimization, how it will be used in the slogan later, and what name will resonate with people. Her eyes shine, her voice is strong, her face is illuminated. She's energized, focused, and confident.

"We did it! PEN.net is available." She frowns. "Umm… A .org is better. We'll fix it later."

I haven't had this much fun since… I can't remember. Let's go celebrate."

"Did John Henry smuggle champagne, too?"

"No, but that's not a bad idea."

We walk to the recreation room and grab a couple of kombucha bottles to toast our new dream.

9 - The Date

A heavy afternoon silence disrupts my concentration. Outside, even birds and insects are napping. I initiate a video chat with Daniel. He's at his desk, dressed in a silver-gray suit, which pairs so well with his green eyes. Suits always outline his confidence and add to his elegant allure. He just finished a meeting with the London office—his trips have been re-placed with video meetings.

Five weeks of seeing each other only through a camera. A digital relationship is like staring at ice cream through a store window. Nevertheless, our dates are still the only joy in this desert.

He comes on the screen, leaning back on his chair. His face still bears a veil of sadness. The frown lines are deeper; he struggles to keep his posture straight. High stacks of papers are piled on the desk. On one hand, I feel his pain. On the other, I wish he didn't miss her so much. Later, I will blame myself for this childish jealousy. It's a strange cognitive dissonance that leaves me frustrated and confused.

"I have some exciting news," I blurt.

"I know. You're leaving next week."

"True. But there's more. Remember my friend Donna? She wants to start an organization to help connect patients with health providers and create clinics similar to Años Mejores to teach people the MicroRiche diet."

"Will you be a part of this venture?"

"Don't have all the details yet, but I might have to move to California."

"California?" He lowers his gaze. "So, when's your departure day?"

"I'm meeting with Dr. Hidalgo tomorrow and should be on my merry way on Tuesday."

"I don't want you to take the bus. I'll ask someone to drive you to the airport or come get you myself."

"I'm ahead of you. Diana, the yoga teacher, will drive me. She's going to visit a friend in San Salvador."

"Bueno. I'll pick you up in Ezeiza. Can you stay a couple of days here?"

"I already have my ticket. I'm spending one night in Buenos Aires and will leave in the morning."

"Let's extend it by one day. I still have to give you a tour of the city. I'll get you a hotel room."

"I already have one. But we can have dinner together."

"You're asking me out on a date? I need to check my schedule." He chuckles.

"You'd better be free if you know what's good for you."

ΛΛΛ

After lunch, I walk to my final appointment with Dr. Hidalgo. The small office is bright today. They have installed LED lights. Dr. Hidalgo sits behind his desk with a wide smile. Either he's happy to see me or he has good news—maybe a little of both.

I sit facing him. My cheeks warm; my knees tingle. I can't deny the sparks between us, but thankfully he's too professional to act upon them and I'm in love with someone else. Psych 101 students can figure this one out. The attention from this handsome doctor reminds me I'm a woman, rather than a cancer patient. More than gratitude, it's a kind of permission to feel attractive instead of defective. I straighten my shoulders and sit with my arms crossed, ready to receive my metabolism analysis.

He opens a binder and starts with illustrations. A sphere labeled The Krebs Cycle has all kinds of arrows moving circularly around it. Vitamins and minerals are attached at different stop points of one arrow and before another one starts. That's what's happening inside my body and how nutrients are metabolized. He puts the sheet next to the one from my first test and shows me all the blocked pathways and how they're now flowing with nothing spilling out. On another page, my antioxidant levels have risen dramatically; my B vitamins are all adequate; I show only a slight copper deficiency, which he says could be iron as well. Iron deficiency is a well-known fact to me because of my heavy menstruation, but not a topic I want to discuss.

As he goes through the pages, something jumps at me. "What's orotic acid?"

He pulls out another sheet of paper. "It's a metabolite of aspartic acid, a byproduct of protein. When it's elevated, it could mean liver damage or a deficiency in magnesium or B vitamins. It also happens when people are undergoing chemotherapy. But yours is completely normal."

He scrolls through the list of biochemistry names and explains what he deems most important for me to know. His face lights up when he comes to another complicated marker, Hydroxyphenyllactate. He shows me the value of the first test and compares it to the latest result.

"You see this metabolite here? It's a pro-oxidative marker. Look how high it was three months ago. It has decreased tremendously. High levels of p-Hydroxyphenyllactate are often associated with carcinogenesis. This is another reason we gave you the high doses of vitamin C."

The more he talks, the more I'm uplifted. His knowledge of biochemistry, his confidence, and the way he looks at me—a certainty in his eyes that I'll be cancer-free—renews my faith in the treatment.

When I tell him about Donna's project to open a similar center in California, his eyes open wider. "That's a great idea. We need more people doing this type of work."

"Will you be available for remote consulting until we find someone locally?"

"Managing this place takes most of my time, but I can provide support until you find the right person." His lips moved as if he wants to add something but stopped himself.

"Can you recommend someone?"

"I'll have to look at my contacts. I do attend the Functional Medicine Conferences and I know some colleagues in the U.S."

He closes my file, hands it to me, and stands. "You're all set. Do you have a ride when you leave tomorrow?"

"Diana is driving me to the airport."

He moves toward me, and this time I don't resist. We exchange a warm hug, knowing we'll probably never see each other again.

I return to my room, pull out my suitcase, and prepare to say goodbye to three months of my life. It's strange how pliable the human mind is. We can get used to anything when we are deprived of choice. I grew accustomed to the isolation, the daily routine of catered meals, and yoga; even fasting became part of this routine and I didn't mind it anymore. A creeping sensation of fatigue climbs my being when I think of resuming life with all its obligations.

The center provided a protective shield from the world's troubles and life's responsibilities. Among patients, there is an honesty rarely seen in other parts of life. They talk freely about their disease, pain, and fears. Regardless of background, social status, or education, our vulnerability makes us all equal.

I text Donna to invite her for a walk. She shows up at my door dressed for a soirée: hair up with curly strands framing her face, pink lipstick, and gray eyeshadow. A fitted navy blue dress accentuates her curves.

"Got a hot date?" I ask.

"Yes! With you."

"Sorry, you're not my type. I like flat chests with a lot of hair."

"Haha! I hired someone to design our website. He asked for pictures of us. So, I need you to take a picture of me."

"Aren't you moving a bit fast?"

"This project is giving me wings. Besides, I dropped five more pounds. I brought this size eight dress with me but didn't really believe I'd fit in it again. Imagine my surprise when I slipped into it eff-ort-less-ly!"

As we walk on the dusty trail, we scout for the best places to take pictures. Enchanted in her new body, Donna strikes a pose at every step. She looks me up and down as if seeing me for the first time. "Hard to believe you're leaving tomorrow."

"I think I've become lazy. After being pampered here, I'm apprehensive about returning to the real world."

"You're not lazy; you're scared. Annie, if your last hour has come, you wouldn't be here. I want you to stop worrying and think about all the wonderful things you and I will accomplish. Our association will go international. You'll deliver talks on TV shows and radio; you'll conduct interviews. Just imagine all the people we'll help."

Her enthusiasm bounces on me like a child on a trampoline, but I remain optimistically cautious— only forty-eight percent of patients in my age group live past the five-year mark with my type of tumor.

"I'll miss you, but not as much as Dr. Hidalgo will. All he has left is the old and ugly."

"Donna!"

"Honey, you're the youngest and most beautiful person in this place. Everyone knows it."

ΛΛΛ

I wake up early and perform a last check of the bubble I'm about to leave. I close the door, wheel my suitcase, and walk to the breakfast table to partake in the last meal with the little group that's been a family for the past three months.

The first person who comes to me is Julie. A pearly white smile on her face is as shiny as jewelry. Her eyes brim with tears as she hugs me. "Thank you, Annie," she whispers. "Can you believe I went running yesterday?"

Her mother interrupts. "If you ever come to Belgium, you have a home." She hands me her contact information.

Others congratulate me and wish me well.

I tip Stefani and Sonia. I shake Chef Laora's hand and thank her for the fabulous meals.

Donna lifts my bag and walks me to the car.

"Travel safe. We'll start working as soon as we're both home and settled. I'll see you soon, okay?" We hug as we push back tears.

^^^

I have little memory of my trip here when Daniel dropped me off the first time. I was so exhausted, I slept most of the way. As Diana drives through a variety of vegetation, desert flowers, and blooming cacti, my eyes sweep the landscape to take a mental image of its beauty. What a wonderful vacation it would be to explore Jujuy!

To kill time, Diana and I exchange our life stories. She talks about growing up in poverty with an absentee father and how she got pregnant as a teenager, followed by a miscarriage.

"At the time, I was glad the baby knew it landed in the wrong place and fled."

"Did you have other children?"

"I never found the right man. But I found the right job. I love what I do, but it does limit my chances for a relationship. What's your story, Annie?"

"Nothing special. I was adopted when I was a baby by the most wonderful parents. I've lived a charmed life. But, one day everything changed and I don't know if it'll ever change back."

The mere mention of cancer mutes people and makes them dissociate. She regains her voice and our conversation turns toward what we have in common: Años Mejores. Diana has fond memories of all the patients who have visited the center over the years. Her stories of different patients, the success of the center, and her love for yoga get us to the airport. We hug with our masks on and she wishes me luck.

I check my suitcase and take the escalator to the gate. I follow a small group of travelers but keep my distance. Crowds are suffocating; like a prisoner who discovers freedom again, I need more breathing room.

I sit facing the long glass wall and gaze at the desert

beyond the parked airplanes. I pull out my phone to communicate with Daniel, but he's ahead of me. He sent emojis of kisses, hugs, and different celebration themes. I reply, but he's offline. After five weeks of video meetings, today feels like a first date, but the excitement of seeing him is overshadowed by the omnipresence of Nina. A plane speeds on the runway and takes off. I follow it until it disappears in the sky.

In most of our online dates, Daniel looked tired and, at times pensive or withdrawn. My clinical education tells me we need to separate for a while so he can process the emotions of loss. But when I mentioned it to him, he refused to hear it. The conversation was heavy and still resonates in my mind.

"How would that help? I'll miss two people instead of one."

"I'd like to make the process easy on you. When you've been a caregiver for years, you develop a routine, a way of life that revolves around that person. Your happiness and peace of mind depend on her comfort and happiness."

"You're right. I feel empty. Kinda lost. I need to get used to being on my own." He hesitates, as he always does when he's afraid of hurting my feelings. "I have to be honest, Annie... I miss her terribly."

And there it was. The confirmation of my fears; the escalation of jealousy. Unintended betrayal. I loved someone who loved someone else.

His eyes shined with tears. We stared at the computer screen in silence before we pretended we had other things to do. We ended the video with his usual "Love you tons, miss you miles." I was the first to click *End.*

We continued our weekly online dates. While he progressively became cheerful, I felt cold and distant. I'm unsure how I'll react to his presence today, so I refused to let him pick me up at the airport. I found a small hotel in Buenos Aires and asked him to come at 7:00 p.m. I wanted to be picked up like any ordinary date. We've had none of those. Our relationship jumped from online to being together without anything in between.

I land in Buenos Aires around 1:00 p.m. Eager to practice my baby Spanish, I ask for information about getting a cab.

"Por favor, donde esta el taxi?"

A small woman, barely visible behind her mile-high pile of suitcases, yells at me from twenty feet away.

"You want a taxi?"

"Yes, please."

"Follow me. I need one, too."

"Thank you."

"Are you American?" she asks.

"I am."

"I went to the States only once, when I was fifteen. I went to Disney World in Florida."

Why are all these people going to Florida?

I say, "Your English is perfect."

"I work for a European company, so I speak English every day."

The nice Samaritan puts me in a cab. I hand the driver a written note with the address of the hotel. He replies in Spanish, but way too fast for me to make anything of it. We both smile and nod.

Quaint Duque Hotel is located a couple of miles from Daniel's house––at least, that's what he said. My room is spacious, with a king-size bed, a small desk, and a chair. I step on the balcony overlooking the pool and luscious green gardens. The hotel is modest but has all the ingredients for romance.

I change and head downstairs to ask the concierge about the best shopping places in town. Buenos Aires is the fashion capital of South America.

As soon as I exit the elevator, I hear the usual WhatsApp chirp.

Hola, mi amor.

Si, como estas?

Are you sure you want to continue in Spanish? he writes with laughing emojis.

No, I prefer to pretend I'm a helpless woman in your country.

In other words, you did not study that hard. How was your trip? Are you at the hotel?

All good. I'm about to go out to explore the city.

Are you sure you don't want us to meet earlier?

Positive.

Annie, this is so silly.

We're meeting in four hours! I want to surprise you.

As you wish!

The concierge recommends only one department store: Galeria Pacifico. His enthusiasm and praise of the place are so compelling I don't ask for any other reference. He points at the facade on a brochure to show me how European it looks.

"It started as the headquarters of the first French department store in Paris: Le Bon Marché, built in 1838. This building was supposed to be their Argentinian headquarters," he says with a thick, sexy Spanish accent as he hands me the brochure of the luxurious mall.

He opens a small map of the inside of the building. "Here, you will find all you want. Beautiful place to spend un afternoon." He points at a food court with a fountain and fashion boutique names from around the world.

The doorman calls a cab for me; he tells the driver where to take me, and he waves us goodbye as we drive off.

The cab driver drops me in front of a tall building at the corner of Cordoba and Florida streets. The entrance is marked by a half-moon-shaped logo of the mall that sits on tall glass-and-bronze doors under a two-story glass facade beneath a stone arch—a flawless composition of classical and modern architecture.

Unlike regular malls serving as commercial districts, Galeria Pacifico takes shopping to another level. Ornate walls with carvings, decorative ironwork, and frescos on vaulted ceilings connect art to fashion.

A boutique catches my eye as I approach the fountain: Versailles. A beautifully decorated French boutique with flowers, long vases, stylish furniture, and sexy blonde mannequins staring at me through the glass window; I can't resist such an invitation.

The saleswoman greets me with a bright smile and presents me with a basket of chocolate. "Vous parlez français ou Espagnol?" she asks.

"English," I reply in a worried tone.

"Oh, mi colleague can help. She speak French and inglés. Nadine!" she calls to the back of the store.

A young woman in her early twenties comes to the rescue. With a melodious accent, she asks "Ello, how can I elp yoo?"

"I have a date and I'm looking for something formal, sexy, yet elegant."

"I know exactly what you need. Please come with me," says the beautiful, trilingual fashion expert.

I follow her to a long line of dresses, short skirts, blouses, and more mannequins posing in elegant nightgowns. She immediately pulls out a soft pink sheath with elbow-long sleeves.

"Zis is perfect for your complexion. But if yoo want to showcase your beautiful red hair, yoo could use a light scarf, like zis one, to put a distance between ze color of yor hair and ze dress." She pulls a light blue scarf with a few pink and green motifs and hands it to me.

"If yoo don't like pink, it comes in white and red as well. But pink is neutral. It's elegant without making a statement. Just feminine, happy, and discreetly sexy."

Nadine shows me to the fitting room and waits for me while I put on the pink dress and scarf. The expression on her face says "Mission Accomplished" when I come out. She makes me turn, pulls softly on my hips to smooth out panty lines, flattens the shoulders to even them out, adjusts the scarf, and with a smile that brightens her face, she asks for my opinion.

"Do yoo like? Yoo look like a model. So beautiful."

After getting over the shock of the price tag— never paid four hundred dollars for a dress before—I walk fast to the cashier before more temptation grabs a hold of my wallet. I hand over my credit card and close my eyes. After I collect the beautiful bag holding the dress, I leave the mall to return to the hotel. I have two hours to get ready. Knowing Daniel, he'll arrive much earlier than planned.

Once in the room, I shower, style my hair into a bun, and dress my face with light makeup: some blush, mascara to shape my eyelashes, and finish with pink lipstick to match the dress. The same butterflies of a first date flutter under my skin.

I'm still apprehensive. Nothing I've read about grieving has prepared me for this situation: being with a man who's missing another woman.

But this evening is mine. I want it to be the best date we've had up to now. I feel healthy, and according to Nadine, I'm stunning in the dress. All those wonderful meals at Años Mejores, the megadoses of vitamin C, and the stress-free days put a glow on my face.

Fifteen minutes to seven, the concierge rings to announce I have a visitor. I give permission to let him come up. One last glance in the mirror. I adjust my hair, take a deep breath, and open the door.

He's standing before me. I almost swoon. We close the door and he moves slowly toward me like a lion sizing up his prey. I stand frozen at first, then give in to the warm, tight squeeze of his arms. My fingers run over his hair.

"Let me look at you," he says as he steps back while holding both my hands. "You look so..."

"It's the dress."

"It's you." He brings me closer and undoes my hair as he kisses me. "I have to stop or we'll never make it to dinner."

"I'm not really hungry."

"You need to eat. Let's go. I have a reservation at a Brazilian restaurant near the hotel. We can walk there. Most restaurants in Buenos Aires are closed since the pandemic. This one serves mainly as an annex to the hotel's restaurant, for when people want to dine outside the hotel but don't want to travel far."

I'd rather make love.

We walk to Açúcar e Coco, a small restaurant with a teal green awning and pink window frames. The spread-out seating respects social distancing. It's a big restaurant, but the menu's restricted. He asks if I can tolerate alcohol and insists I try a famous Brazilian cocktail. He motions to the waiter, a tall man with bronze skin and a ponytail.

"Um Caipirinha com Maracuja, por favor!"

"You speak Portuguese?"

"Enough to order cocktails."

After the waiter leaves, we resume our conversation, but he's jittery; his hands fidget with the napkin and rearranging the silverware.

"There's something on your mind," I say.

"Nina left something for you."

I swallow to moisten my dry throat. "Me? How did she know about me?"

"I told her."

"Why would you do that?"

"She knew. Call it a woman's intuition, or maybe she saw something in my demeanor."

"Was she upset?"

He bows his head and smiles in a manner I find condescending. "Nooo. One afternoon, she asked to see me. I entered the room, and she gestured with her eyes for me to sit close to her. She hadn't done that in two years. Then she asked, 'Are you happy, Daniel?' She looked at me with her usual wicked smile when she was hiding something. I said yes. Then she asked, 'What's her name?' I was speechless. 'You don't have to worry about my feelings. Was the plan,' she said. Then everything became clear: the irrational demand for a divorce, the refusal to let me get close to her... She set me up."

"I see. How generous of her."

"I asked how she knew. She said, 'I know *you*.' So, I told her your name, and she looked at me with a mixture of love and sadness. I can't explain it. She said, 'Annie? It's a noble name. Giving you up was harder than giving up my body, but it was the right thing to do.'"

"That's quite a woman."

"She was gone two days later."

I don't think there is a word to describe the combination of anger, shock, and sadness. Maybe rage. No, not strong enough. If someone were to draw my face, I'd have bulging red eyes, a wide-open mouth blowing flames, and tubes of smoke escaping from my ears. Did she engineer this entire relationship? She gets credit for watching over his happiness and I'm a puppet in her game—a tool in her strategy. Before I digest the news, he hands me an envelope.

"She was very organized and methodical. She wrote each of us a letter. This one's for you."

Instead of punching him in the face, I clench my jaw and tuck the envelope into my purse. How far will she push this superwoman act? This isn't class or dignity. It's about control and greed. She wants to anchor her presence in our relationship forever.

The waiter puts our drinks on the table. I grab the glass and gulp half of it down. It's heavenly. Nothing tastes better than passion fruit and rum. But it doesn't quench the flames of rage.

"This is also her plan? To poison us from the grave?" I almost shout.

"What do you mean?"

"I wanted this evening to be about you and me, not the three of us."

"Why are you twisting this?"

"She had no intention of giving you up. She wanted to make sure you admire and think about her every single day. This is pure manipulation."

"I don't like where this is going."

"Neither do I. Maybe you should find yourself another superwoman who's into sharing."

I throw the napkin on the table and storm out of the

restaurant before the mascara melts on my face. Once I'm far enough, I look back. He's sitting with his arms crossed on the table and his head down. I walk to the hotel, wiping streams of mascara. I rush through the lobby, avoiding eye contact with anyone. *Shit! I have to wait for the elevator.* I hope he doesn't walk behind me and find me disintegrated. I pace until the elevator doors open.

I dart out of the elevator at my floor, into my room, and straight to the bathroom to wash my face. I stare at the mirror to remember the woman I used to be. *Why did I react with such fury?* I've never experienced such jealousy. It's an impulse that penetrates the heart like a sword, bursting out the other side like a dragon's breath and scorching everything in its path. I pat my face dry, sit on the bed, and try to make sense of my rage. *Damn! Another symptom of brain surgery.* I thought I was done with that.

I pull the letter from my purse and hold it on my lap. At first, I wanted to tear it into pieces, but I can't resist the temptation of hearing Nina's voice. I open the folded page to discover this woman who's been haunting me for months. Her weak voice becomes alive through the ink. I read and sob.

Dear Annie,

By the time you read this, I will have left this world. It's with both joy and sorrow that I write to you. I write with sorrow because I'm leaving behind all that I love. I write with joy because I know Daniel will not be alone. He's a wonderful man, a devoted husband, and the best father a child can hope for.

You must wonder how I could let go of such a man. It wasn't easy, but when doctors told me I was at the end-of-life stage, I released Daniel so he could find happiness with someone else. I didn't want him to be alone after I'm gone. So, I'm glad he's met you and you make him happy. He's been more relaxed and a better caregiver since he met you.

He's an easy man to love and live with. However, he doesn't like arguing. He will shut down and walk away if a conversation gets heated. It's best you go to him for a reconciliation, as he won't know how to come out of the silence. He's a workaholic, so you'll have to organize activities around him and plan vacations to get him away from his computer.

About our daughter Tanya, and this is the hardest part for me. My disability has profoundly affected her and made her grow up faster than most children. She's smart, sweet, beautiful, and very close to her father. It's with much pain and sadness that I have to leave her at such a delicate age, but I tried to hold on to life until life could no longer hold on to me.

Even though I wanted Tanya to have as normal a childhood as possible, she wanted to help care for me. This has strengthened our bond, but she did not socialize much with her peers. She needs to be reminded to attend social activities with people her age and engage in hobbies. She likes to paint, enjoys theater, and of course, loves animals. I hope you'll encourage her in these activities and help her grow into a confident woman.

Tanya knows you exist, and I told her to support both of you. However, she's a teenager and I cannot predict how all this will affect her. I hope some of the love you have for Daniel will spill over to Tanya so you'll have the patience to accommodate her behavior, if any. She may resent you at first, as is expected, but if you give her time and space to get to know you, you'll find her a wonderful child.

Please focus on your relationship, the future you will build together, and how you can make each other happy. If Daniel loves you, you must be a special person. You shouldn't feel guilty either. Life is a game and we all take turns to play. This is your turn. Enjoy every minute of it.

I'm trusting you with what I love most. I wish you the best life has to offer.

Irena

This is not at all what I expected. As I drown in tears, I feel so many emotions: sadness, anger, fear, remorse. All the anguish and pain of the last months combine into a muddy, sticky ball that weighs in my mid-section. As I try to make sense of it all, I hear a timid knock on the door. I rush to the bathroom to clean my face again.

I open the door and we stand in silence without eye contact.

Head down, he says, “May I come in please?”

I let him in and we sit on the bed with the weight of the air pressing down on us.

“Can you help me understand what just happened?”

My voice quivers. “I planned a romantic evening for the two of us. I didn’t want another woman intruding.”

“I’m sorry. I’m new at this. I didn’t realize it was inappropriate.”

I lean toward him to put my head on his shoulder and he surrounds me with his arm.

“It was such a shock to learn she knew about me. I felt like a pawn in a game. I read the letter… You’re right. She’s the type of person everyone would want as a friend.” I pause to release the heaviness in my chest. “It's sad that someone had to be sacrificed for my happiness.”

“Now that’s the Annie I know and love.” He kisses my head. “I’m glad you read the letter. It was a tremendous effort for her to produce it. The nurse said she could barely talk when she dictated them.”

“I still worry I can’t make you as happy as she did.”

“You already do! You’re beautiful, smart, funny, accomplished. Having you in my life is like winning the lottery.”

“Call me old fashioned, but I couldn’t bear the thought of you with another woman, even after I’m dead.”

“We don’t have to worry about that,” he whispers in my hair.

“Your wife is so strong, wise, and near perfect…”

“It wasn’t always like that. She had the same insecurities most women have. She complained about her nails constantly. Do you know how much I care about nails?”

“I guess not much.”

"She wouldn't wear a bikini because she thought her breasts were too small. I told her I was a leg man, not a boob man."

"She had nice legs?"

He points his finger at me and winks. "Not falling for it!"

My hesitation fades; my coldness melts away. Like a compulsion, I want to be closer to him, the kind of closeness that confirms with certainty he's mine and it's right. I wrap my legs around his hips and sit on his lap facing him with my arms around his shoulders. I let myself be absorbed by the silence. My fingers furrow through his hair, holding his face in the nook of my neck. His hands run over my back. The days of absence are sealed by our closeness and the previous hours are erased by the warmth of our kisses. Interlaced, our bodies use their own intimate language to communicate, apologize, and forgive. Then, he cups my face with his hands.

"Annie, you should never doubt my love for you. It scared me when you walked out of the restaurant." He raises my hand to make me look at my fingers. "Which one of these would you say is irrelevant?"

"Come again?"

"It's the same with love. Every person you love occupies their own space in your heart. There is no ladder of importance or seniority status. Every time you love, it's different, often stronger and deeper because you've gained more experience and have a better grasp of the fragility of happiness."

"How many years did you spend in Tibet?"

"Enough to know you're precious and I'm never letting you go."

Our lips meet again. I take off into space like weightless puffs of dandelion seeds in search of fertile soil. My hair is spread over his face; he sweeps it back, kisses my forehead, and breathes into my neck, "We'll get through this, but we have to stay together."

Like a cool breeze after a hot summer day, tears roll

down my cheeks and it's all peaceful again. He kisses me softly all over my face and whispers in Spanish, "Te amo como Dios ama a quienes lo adoran."

Although a little more syrupy than I can handle, it's still good to hear. We stand up. The pink dress falls slowly to the floor. Our hands move freely over each other. His bronze skin contrasts with my milky white complexion. I wrap my arms around his neck and lose myself in the beauty of our love. He lets me lead, but gently takes control and explores my most intimate parts and ignites them into bouquets of fireworks that explode into millions of colors—red, green, with gold dominating, like Klimt's *The Kiss*.

I exorcised the ghost; I claimed my territory; I'm home at last. It's an intense awareness of belonging and wishing to forever stay.

He props himself up and leans against the backboard, supported by pillows. I lie next to him and let my hand wander over his chest as my fingers revel in the warmth of his skin.

"You're a boob man in the closet."

"Coming out is liberating."

I giggle. "I'm happy for you."

He picks up the phone. "I have an idea. Let's order room service. Are you hungry?"

"Not really."

"You need to eat." He opens the menu and orders for both of us. I'm vegan, after all.

10 - The Wait is Over

I wake to rain pearling the hotel windows. It's too early for the sun to rise, but the grey sky looks warm and cozy, like a hiding place. I pull up the covers and snuggle next to him. I have not felt this kind of serenity in months, like a sailor who comes home after a long journey at sea.

When he opens his eyes, I say, "Buenos días, amor!"

"¿Como pasaste la noche?" He wraps his arms around me and nibbles on my neck.

"Take it easy now! Only been here one day."

"Practically a Porteña." He scoops my body on top of his. "I was asking if you slept well."

"I didn't sleep."

"Why not?"

"I'm too happy. I wanted to live the night."

"You can always take a nap later."

"Like you'll let me take a nap."

"Is there such a thing as an active nap?" A knock at the door interrupts our embrace. "I ordered breakfast last night."

A waiter wheels in a table with a basket of pastries, a coffee carafe, and a teapot. As tempting as the fresh croissants are, I'm not hungry.

I pour myself a cup of tea. "You know, I think the best weight loss program is happiness."

"Whoever coined the expression 'living on love and water' has probably done it." He fills his coffee cup and pushes the basket toward me. "This is vegan. They're made with margarine instead of butter and dark chocolate has no dairy."

"I'm so relieved," I say, shaking my head and laughing. "I'll save a croissant for later."

"I know your secret. You don't sleep. You don't eat. You're a Goddess." He bites into a pain au chocolate and hands me a brochure. "What would you like to do today?"

"I want to go to San Telmo. I heard it's a nice bohemian city with art galleries and a flea market."

"Technically, not a city. Buenos Aires is divided into

barrios. San Telmo is one of them."

"Which barrio do you live in?"

He looks at me with his usual half smile when he wants to avoid answering a question. "I already told you. You forgot."

"Tell me again."

"When you're ready, I'll give you a tour of my neighborhood."

End of conversation. I'm not ready to see the home he shared with his wife; I don't want ghosts haunting our last day together.

I take my cup of tea to the window to watch Buenos Aires wake up. Cars, people, and bikes move hurriedly around each other, rushing to their destination. On the horizon, the sun is piercing the clouds.

"The flea market in San Telmo is enormous. There are also concerts in the street, mimes, and painters. I have an acquaintance who owns a vegan restaurant there. He makes the most amazing empanadas. We'll stop there for lunch."

"I doubt they're as good as the ones I've had at Años Mejores."

"Eduardo is a fantastic chef. There aren't many vegan-friendly restaurants in Buenos Aires. It's hell for vegans!"

"Maybe I should show you my new culinary skills."

"Hmmm... a gorgeous woman who cooks vegan? I may not let you leave."

By the time we're ready to leave the hotel, the sun is shining bright, turning the rain puddles into mirrors. The concierge warned me about the weather. Days often start with small thunderstorms in the early morning hours, followed by sunshine later in the day. The autumn sky is a crisp blue with soft sunlight drawing our shadows as we explore the most European city of the southern hemisphere.

ΛΛΛ

The day in Buenos Aires flew by at lightning speed. We

walked through crowds of masked people, dancing and singing, Daniel squeezed my hand and my soul sank into the velvety warmth of our kisses. Everything swirled in the color of joy and hope.

The bumpy landing at Dulles Airport jolts me out of my reverie.

After three months in Argentina, stepping off the airplane drops me violently back into my world like landing in the jungle without a parachute. I'm light and hollow as I pass through Customs. Robotically trudging through the noisy, crowded hallways to the luggage carousel, I collect my suitcase, exit the airport, and hail a cab.

The driver furrows through traffic along the boring Jersey barriers, toll plazas, and traffic lights, while my mind wanders off to Buenos Aires until he drops me off in front of my door. Spring has arrived in Virginia. Fuchsia azalea blooms, yellow daffodils, red tulips, and delicate white and pink dogwoods cast a festive ambiance on the neighborhood. I pause before opening the door and re-entering my life.

A basket of fruit and a greeting card welcome me when I step inside the house. Sweet Tina. A cascade of white blooms hangs from the orchid; the snake plant looks taller; my mail is neatly stacked on the table. I quickly inspect the house. Everything is the way I left it. The silence and emptiness wrap around me and press me down.

After about an hour of contemplation, I peel myself off the couch and move to the bathroom for a hot shower to wash away the gloom. As soon as I get out of the bathroom, the phone beeps in a steady stream: WhatsApp from Daniel; text and email from my parents and a few friends. A warm sensation of finding home again replaces the burden of loneliness.

Daniel: *Hola, mi amor, have you made it home safely? Miss you.*

Mom: *Let us know you got home okay.*

Tina: *Hey, Annie, welcome back! Happy hour tomorrow? I want to hear more about your Argentinian adventure.*

Donna: *Hope the trip home wasn't too tiring. AM feels empty without you.*

Once I reply to everyone, I hit the grocery store for a new shopping experience. No more bacon or turkey cutlets; cheese is a distant memory. I push my cart to the produce section to fill it with beets, celery, lettuce, cabbage, kale, jicama, and seasonal fruit, then turn to the "lean protein" section and fill up on bags of chickpeas, beans, nuts, and seeds. As I wait in line at the cashier, I snap a picture of the cart and text it to Daniel. "Mira me!"

Ron is waiting for me next to the azalea bush. He empties the last content of the beer can in his mouth and crumples it in his hand.

"You're back from your sabbatical."

I pull grocery bags out of the trunk. Ron offers to help carry them.

"It's nice to be home."

"Missed you, sweetheart. Neighborhood was boring while you were gone."

"Thanks for keeping an eye on the house."

"Always!" he says as he drops the bags in front of the door. "Take care of yourself, okay?"

It's official! I'm home.

I put away the groceries but don't feel like cooking. The heavy weight of loneliness crashes down on me. I settle for a coconut yogurt topped with raspberries and pumpkin seeds. I listlessly scroll through movie trailers on the laptop.

/\ /\ /\

Monday at 9:00 a.m., I call Dr. Drapeau's office to schedule the long-awaited MRI. Part of me wants to postpone indefinitely; the other part wants to know immediately. The receptionist confirms the doctor will send the referral to the imaging center as a priority, and he'll see me after he receives the results. I haven't told anyone about the appointment. If my life is about to end, I'll need time to absorb the news before sharing it.

A cheerful voice answers the phone at the imaging center and schedules me for a noon slot. The wait is over. Nothing more to do.

I arrive early at the imaging center. A young woman named Jocelyn greets me with a soft voice that blends into the room's pastel colors. She hands me a clipboard with a stack of forms to fill out.

The waiting room is spacious, with modern light fixtures and large paintings; green plants fill every corner. Vases and bowls are strategically positioned on flat surfaces. The decor gives the room a hotel lobby feel—anything to distract us from the reason for our visit. But nothing can overshadow the despair. These walls have seen many diminished lives and threatened futures; they are the gate of doom. Many people walk out of here with their lives changed forever; a few walk out… never to return.

I sit next to a bald man in his mid-forties who's whispering something to a teenage boy. Facing me, a woman with a pale face and wispy hair is filling out forms, and next to her, another woman, probably in her thirties, is texting. Cancer hits at random and without discrimination.

After I circle a list of "NOs" next to more medical conditions and provide my height and weight, I sign and return the clipboard to Jocelyn, who directs me to wait for the technician.

Chris, a slender man with a lab coat, calls my name. He takes me to another room for more questions. He goes over the safety form I just filled out. Can this go any slower? I want to scream. But he has to do his job methodically. I'm just another name on his roster. This is the part that I have not come to terms with: being someone's job. I answer his questions, smile, and choke on my frustration.

"Is this your first MRI?"

"I had one a few months ago."

He finally hands me a robe and socks and orders me to take off all my clothes and jewelry in the locker room.

The exam room is cold, white, and sterile. Lots of drawers and containers on the countertop filled with an assortment of medical supplies—all white. Clenching my fists, I shout internally, *I'm not supposed to be here!* Unable to come out of my mouth, the rage bubbles into water through my eyes. I remind myself to stay in control and put palms to eyes to press back the tears.

"Is the room too bright?" Chris asks, ever so attentive.

I position myself on the exam table, which Chris raises using a control panel on the front of the machine, and I find myself before a giant mouth about to swallow my body. He places a cushion beneath my knees and covers me with a blanket. I put my head in a cradle as he goes over the procedure a final time.

"Once the scan starts, you'll need to keep still so we get clear images. In about fifteen minutes, I'll come in to inject the contrast with a small needle stick through your arm, wherever I can find a vein."

"For you, I'll grow some."

"That's what they all say." I got a small rise out of him, but he quickly goes back to business. "You may feel a cold sensation going through your arm. Some people feel nothing."

He hands me a little rubber ball hooked to the table by a flexible plastic tube. "If you need to talk to me, feel uncomfortable, need to scratch, sneeze, just squeeze right here," he says, pointing at the ball.

He secures the headphones over my ears and a large piece of equipment reminiscent of a catcher's mask over my head. It covers the head and face with a little cut-out window for the eyes. The handles snap into the cradle. The combination of the coil snapping into place and my headphones make it a snug fit. *I have to stay like this for…?* I pant.

"You need to breathe slowly and as quietly as possible," Chris advises in my ears. "Would you like some music now?"

"Sure. The Magic Flute."

"You got it."

A few seconds later, Mozart is comforting me.

He pushes a button on the remote control, and the table enters the tube. I don't remember how I made it through last time. Being squeezed inside this tunnel, I'm afraid of suffocating. I breathe slowly, as instructed—keep those images crisp. I fill my mind with the happy times I had with Daniel. His gentle touch, his warm smile, the sunshine in his eyes when he looks at me, and his soothing voice when he says he loves me. Those memories drown the thumping and buzzing of the sci-fi creature holding me in its mouth.

Chris' voice coming through the headphones interrupts my daydream. "I'm about to give you the contrast." He comes in and slides the table partway. I extend my arm and feel a sharp pinch. He advises me not to move my head, then I'm swallowed again.

I shiver beneath the blanket. I want to move my head or rotate my body, but pressing on the rubber ball will delay the procedure. The faster it goes, the sooner I'll be out. Remembering Diana's instructions, I focus on my breathing and return to images of Buenos Aires.

Finally, the machine stops shouting. The ensuing silence sounds louder—but only for a moment. The table slides out from the scanner. Chris removes the coil and the headphones before lowering the table.

"That wasn't so bad. You did great."

I thank him as he walks me to the locker room, where I change into my costume of a healthy woman about to be lost in the crowd.

In the parking lot, I start the car, but I'm unable to move. My legs are limp; my head is empty. I stare at the oak tree in the distance, then back at the clock on the dashboard. In a few hours, I will know if the end is near. I breathe deep to relax my nerves and order my muscles to move.

On the way home, I meander through the back roads to kill time. What a strange concept! Time: our most precious commodity, yet people always want to waste it. I may not have enough to spare, so why not enjoy these hours instead of killing them?

I park in Reston Town Center to find a restaurant. A quick online search shows a vegan restaurant nearby called Kale and Berry—a cozy, comfortable place to dine solo.

As I walk the two blocks to the restaurant, a calm sensation runs over me. Fear and anxiety are when there is hope and one can take action. My gaze stops on a rabbit hopping out of the bushes. Without fear or hesitation, he crosses the street a few feet away and looks at me once he reaches the other side. I smile. This little creature had a goal and pursued it with resolve and determination. A glow of hope shines inside me. There is still a chance things will turn out well.

The restaurant has four tables and no waiters; just a cashier behind a large glass window who takes orders. He's a short man with round eyes; a blue mask is stretched over his puffy face and his bald head glistens under the fluorescent light. I lean to the left to read the menu on the blackboard behind him. After placing my order, I grab a bottle of water from the fridge and choose a table near the window. People who walk by don't notice the restaurant. Those with jobs are in a hurry. Young people walk and text and women slow their pace to search their purses. By the end of the day, many of them will receive news that will disrupt their lives forever. Others will rejoice after receiving a long-awaited phone call. Dreams, plans, schedules can change in an instant. We have so little control over our lives, yet we pretend we own it. But without that naive insouciance that makes people oblivious at funerals, the world would not go around.

I pick up the food when the cashier calls my name and return to the table. I run a fork through the vibrant colors to incorporate the dressing, but they fail to stimulate my appetite.

I check email, browse social media, click on likes, and comment. After about an hour, I only ate a couple of bites; I ask for a to-go box.

The tires slowly roll on the tarmac as I drive to the doctor's office, consuming the last minutes of oblivion in a space where everything is still possible. I'm lightheaded and a knot has formed in my mid-section. If nothing has changed, there is nowhere else to go. I clench the steering wheel as my eyes wander to the blooming shrubbery along the beltway, which is usually packed at this hour, but not today. Without traffic, I arrive early at the hospital. Dead woman walking.

Dr. Drapeau sits with the same posture and empty expression as when I first met him. His silver hair is neatly combed back, and his blue eyes peer beneath bushy eyebrows. He greets me with that cold and detached professional formula: "How are you?"

"Depends on what you have to say," I answer.

"How're you feeling today? Any problems with memory, fatigue?"

"No, I actually feel very healthy."

He lifts his eyes from the manila folder. "I see you turned down treatment."

"The treatment would extend my life by two to five years, with horrendous side effects."

He frowns and turns to his computer.

This is bad news. I put my hands on my shaking knees. The knot in my stomach is bigger.

With his back still turned, he manipulates the monitor and faces me. "I received the images just a few minutes ago."

He displays the black and white ovals that are my brain cut into slices: the cauliflower-like cerebellum, the two distinct lobes, and a white blob on the upper left lobe.

"It looks like the tumor is gone. There is no activity. Do you see the white splotch here? That's a little edema as the body tries to absorb the dead material." He switches pictures and shows me the first MRI. "In this one, we can see the tumor, much larger and active. There is blood supply all around it. But here, there is no tumor, just the surgery scar and edema, which will dissipate over time."

"Are you saying I'm cancer-free?"

"Not exactly. The tumor is gone, but it could grow back. Since you did not receive any treatment, there could be cancerous cells somewhere else in the body. Just not detectable at this time."

"But that tumor is gone, right?"

"Yes, the residual matter we could not remove with surgery seems to have dissolved. I recommend we repeat the MRI in six months."

"Any idea how it dissolved? Have you seen this in other patients?"

"I haven't had any patients turn down treatment. In your case, I'd expect the tumor to grow, not shrink. You're lucky."

"Well, it's not luck. I've received treatment. It's called the MicroRiche diet along with megadoses of vitamin C."

"Nutrition therapy for cancer has not been investigated—not this type, anyway. But if it's working, keep doing it."

I thank him and leave. A wave of heat climbs my legs and floods my body. Similar to those echoes in movies, the phrase *there is no tumor, there is no tumor...* broadcasts loudly in my mind. I'm confused and lost under the blinding April sun as I search for my car in the vast parking lot.

I turn on the ignition, listen to the radio, and wait for the knot in my stomach to unwind. The guillotine blade is lifted, but even good news requires mental adjustment. I drive home on autopilot. I can't feel the road; I don't read the signs; all I see are those black and white pictures with a white splotch and the same phrase echoing over and over.

I find myself in front of my door. I wave back at Ron who's chatting with another neighbor. I enter the house, put my purse on the console, and plop myself on the couch. What just happened? Is it really over? What if it comes back? What if it's already growing somewhere else? *No!* I shout to myself. Today is a good day. I have to live it before moving on to the next.

I exhale a long breath and feel the tension leaving my

body. I pull out the phone to make some calls, but I'm rudely interrupted. A blue jay stares at me from the patio railing. *"Hurry up with that lunch, human!"* I open the door; he flies away.

"This is a dysfunctional relationship, buddy." I pour some seeds into the flower pot and, as soon as I'm back inside, he lands into the pot and munches away—his beautiful tail waving to the azaleas.

Time to announce the good news. First Daniel, then Donna, and my parents in the evening.

Buenas! R u available for a chat? I text.

Annie, everything good with you?

Everything is FUNtastic!

He picks up at the first ring and I talk before he says hello. "I have the best news of the year. Ready?"

"Don't make me wait."

"I just got the MRI results. The tumor is gone. I am cancer-free!" Repeating the words "cancer-free" intensifies their meaning, as if telling someone else validates the results, like highlighting them on a page.

"That's stupendous! I knew you could beat it!" he says without a hint of surprise, but his voice, erupting with joy, is elevated by more than a few decibels. "I just wish I was there with you. Did you go alone?"

I laugh. "I didn't want any witnesses."

"Seriously, I wish you'd told me. We're in this together, you know." The cheerful voice suddenly changes to a slightly reprimanding one.

"I didn't want anyone to worry." The line goes silent for a few seconds. "I'm still in shock. Everything I've read said there was no escape. So, I didn't believe diet would kill a tumor."

"I've never met anyone with your determination. You're a powerhouse of strength, Annie. I love you so much. When do we get together to celebrate?"

"I may have to fly to Oregon to see my parents first."

He ends the call with his "Love you tons, miss you miles."

Donna is next. I know she's waiting to hear from me, but

is afraid to ask. She also answers the call on the first ring.

"Donna? It's Annie. Guess what?"

"You're pregnant! I knew it." Her loud and jaunty laugh is like a summer breeze.

"I sense a desperation for a godmother position."

"So, am I right?"

"Wrong! I had my MRI today and..."

"Oh my God!" She screams so loud, I pull the phone away from my ear. "You don't have cancer! Oh, honey, I'm so happy for you. I'm telling you, these people know what they're doing!" Her sweet, squeaky voice can cheer a mountain buried in fog.

"Well, things look good for now, but the doctor said it can still come back."

"He doesn't know that. He doesn't understand the treatment we received in this place, either. So, go celebrate! Why burden today with problems of tomorrow, which may never happen, anyway?"

"When are you leaving?"

"Next week. Dr. Hidalgo says I'm cured. Well, he didn't exactly use the word 'cure,' but it's time to go home. I'm ten pounds away from my goal weight and I feel better than I have in fifteen years."

There is another person who needs to know the outcome of the treatment: Dr. Hidalgo. I'm his only brain tumor patient. My results could give hope to someone else. But is this really the reason I want to call him? I opt for an email and copy Karina.

To occupy the two-hour wait before calling my parents, I go for a walk —like stepping into a mikvah, I take my first steps as a cancer-free woman.

ΛΛΛ

"Hey, Mom, can we do a Zoom call?"

"Is everything okay?" My mother can always read me with clarity.

"I want to talk to you and Dad at the same time."

They come on the screen and I talk first. "I had an MRI today. Are you ready for the results?"

"We're ready." My mother sighs.

"There is no tumor in my brain."

My father stares at the screen. My mother sweeps her face with both hands to pull her hair back into a ponytail. She whispers, "Sorry, I just floated out of my body. Can you repeat that?"

"That's right, no more cancer."

"Hallelujah!" she shouts, crossing her hands on her chest.

My father passes his hand over his forehead, raises his eyebrows, and leans back to better absorb the shock. His eyes glisten with tears. "Annie!" He sighs. "This is the best news since man walked on the moon."

"I wouldn't go that far, but it is tremendous." I bring my face closer to the camera.

"When are you coming home?" my mother asks.

My father takes over the conversation to use words my mother couldn't. "It's been months since we've seen you in person. There hasn't been one day we didn't think about you." Then he chokes with tears.

"I know. I miss you, too. I have a lot to do here. But I can come in a couple of weeks."

"Give us a date, and we'll invite Uncle Bob and Aunt Lydia. Aunt Bettie, too; she's been asking about you almost every day."

"Okay, I'll take care of a few things here, and we'll plan a visit."

"Honey, we love you," my father gushes. "We're so proud of the way you handled this whole nightmare."

My mother smiles, tilting her head in agreement, and tells me how much she loves me the way she always does—with advice and reprimand.

"Make sure you get enough sleep and eat well. You look bony. Are you taking any supplements? I can find you a good nutritionist."

"Thanks, Mom. I got a good education in Argentina. I'm all set."

11 - It's a Yes or No Answer

Three months later...

The month of June is probably what inspired the state's slogan, *Virginia is for Lovers*. Warm sunshine gleams on blooming flowers, trees, and shrubs. Dogwoods showcase their pastel colors; azaleas boastfully expose their bloom assortment of blood-red, fuchsia, white, and tropical orange; roses and honeysuckles compete to impregnate the air with their aroma. Mild temperature and plenty of daylight make this month the best time of the year.

Traffic is light today on the way to the airport, and despite having plenty of time, I still speed to arrive sooner. I can push the car but not the clock. Two hours before we reunite. I vibrate with excitement, but anxiety, too. The ghost of Nina always hovering above us. I constantly have to shush the gnawing whispers in the back of my mind. *She's the love of his life. You have him by default.*

As soon as I park, my phone beeps. His plane just landed. Doubts, fear, and Nina's ghost fly away. I rush to the waiting line and glue my eyes on the black rubber doors. A long hour passes as I sort through the cohort of travelers staggering out. The large door panels open and close, teasing me. I vent my frustration with foot tapping and humming beneath my breath each time I see yet another person who's not him. Then he emerges, suitcase in hand and a backpack on his shoulder. It's like discovering him all over again. He walks toward me with measured steps and a beaming smile.

Masks off, we hug and kiss—who knows for how long. We always get lost in each other, but this time we linger in the closeness to erase so much pain, fear, and the long months of waiting. When we finally pull away, shouting and applause erupt behind us. A small group of people approve of our PDA—Daniel bows, smiling. I stand in shock.

We pull up our masks and walk out of the airport.

"What a friendly town. Is this how they welcome visitors?" he asks, amused.

"Only Porteños."

We kiss when we get into the car; we kiss at every red light; I drive with one hand while the other is interlaced with his. I turn into the neighborhood, smile at Ron, who's waving at me with a beer, and pull into the driveway. It's the first time Ron has seen me with a man since I moved in. No doubt he'll quiz me later.

"Isn't it a little early for drinking?" Daniel asks.

"Technically, he's breaking the law."

He chortles. "Alcoholism is illegal?"

"It's illegal to drink outdoors in Virginia."

With his hand on my shoulder, he draws me close to him and whispers, "What *else* is illegal?"

He walks into my townhouse, looks around, lifts his chin, and nods to give it a seal of approval.

"Charming. You're a great decorator."

He examines each family and vacation picture—a few on the wall, a couple of frames on the console. He studies each one the way an investigator searches for clues to penetrate someone's life. I take his hand to lead him to the bedroom and offer him a dresser for his clothes. He pushes the suitcase aside and grabs me by the waist.

"The suitcase can wait."

ΛΛΛ

Three flawless days pass. We sleep late, and wake up late; we visit the Smithsonian, Mount Vernon, and the botanical gardens. He loves growing flowers—a hobby started by his wife. We sample several vegan restaurants in the DC Metro area. He's surprised at how much the city has changed since he attended Georgetown University.

"You know what we should do?"

"Qué?" I reply.

"We should try skydiving sometime."

"Fish swim. Birds fly. Humans walk."

"I'll be holding you. You have to see the world from above. It's magic."

I put his hand on my heart. “I’m already on a high every time we’re together.”

He kisses my forehead. “Tonight, I’m taking you even higher. I found a raw vegan restaurant in Great Falls. Not too far from your house.”

“Raw vegan? Here?”

“Absolutely. It looks upscale, too.”

∧∧∧

The restaurant is a beautifully renovated two-story home. Each table is cozy and dressed in a crisp white tablecloth, topped with a small Grecian vase of flowers. Glass water bottles in vibrant colors—cobalt-blue, ruby-red, amber—add a touch of luxury.

After the waiter seats us, we both order a glass of white wine. Daniel is fidgeting. He readjusts his chair, flips through the menu without reading, and looks at the door. He swallows a gulp of wine, then smiles at me while his eyes say, *I have a secret.*

“Have you ever considered changing your name?” he asks.

“What’s wrong with my name?” I reply, taken aback.

He lifts his shoulders. “Nothing. But Mrs. Lorenzo has a better ring to it.”

“Is that a proposal, Mr. Lorenzo?”

He holds my hands. “How would you like to live in Argentina?”

“Permanently?”

“Til death do us part.”

“In my country, when a man proposes, he drops on one knee and presents the lady with a rock.”

“I have something better than a diamond.”

He pulls out an old pouch with dangling strings on each side. It’s frayed at the bottom corners and the little flowers that used to brighten it have faded. He loosens the double strings, then draws out a small white gold band mounted with a sapphire. The design is reminiscent of the 1930s, an elegant minimalist style, unencumbered with extravagant details. He slips it on my finger, but it's too small. I hold it in my palm and move my hand under the light of the table lamp. It throws sparkles of blue light.

"It's my grandmother's."

"Your grandma was tiny."

"Since this is your first time, you want a big wedding?" he asks.

The words "husband", "wife", "forever", swirl in my mind into ribbons of confusion. I'm grateful for the waiter's interruption to take our order but not enough time to sort my thoughts.

After the waiter leaves, he says, "Annie, I haven't heard a 'yes' yet."

I fill my mouth with wine before I formulate an answer. "I think we need more time."

He scowls. "More time for what? Graduate from high school?"

"I'm not ready. Can you understand that?"

"Sure." He sighs, leaning against the chair. He rounds his back and shoulders and looks down at his lap as he unfolds the napkin. "I understand a *NO* when I hear it."

"It's not that simple."

"It is for me."

"You're not the one uprooting your life. Not to mention learning a new language. I'd need to get licensed, find a job?"

"I thought the most important thing was being together. We'll figure out everything else as we go."

"Sure, as long as you make all the decisions." I swallow another gulp of wine. "Would you have proposed if..." I stop myself and look away.

"What? If I were still married?"

"Precisely. I feel like this relationship is on your terms."

"So... this is about punishing me?"

"Of course not. But why is it always for me to adapt to what *you* want? Why don't you move here? You already speak English and your job is portable."

"I have a teenager to raise. After she's self-sufficient, we can move here if you like. But this isn't about moving, is it?"

"What d'you mean?"

"Annie, you're an intelligent woman. Spanish isn't that hard to learn. What are you not telling me?"

Rushing blood warms my face. The rash on my neck flares up; words stick in my dry mouth. I wrap my hands around the stem of the wine glass and stare at its content.

Holding my chin, he lifts my face. "Annie, look at me."

I clench my jaw to prevent words from leaking out. This is the information I did not want to share with anyone.

"The doctor said there's a good chance the cancer will return. We'll know for sure in two to five years."

"So, in the meantime, we put our lives on hold? If there is a risk you'll get sick again, then we should get married even sooner. Why waste time? I don't want us to be separated again."

Perhaps one of his most admirable qualities. When he's ready, his decision is firm. Only, I don't know if it's a quality I'll enjoy or a source of conflict that'll come between us.

"I also want to start this business venture with Donna."

"Why can't you work remotely and travel back when necessary?"

"I'm her right hand and co-owner. She needs me to do a lot of the presentations, meet with investors, get the business off the ground. I may have to move to California if it takes off."

"I'm sure you'll be very successful. There'll be nothing distracting you. But who will you share this success with when you get there?"

"Daniel..."

"I don't want to discuss this anymore. Let's go." He gestures to the waiter to bring the check. The muscles in his face are tense; he lowers his head and rests his closed fists on the table.

When the waiter comes to our table, he looks at the

untouched food, examines our faces, and asks in shock, "What's wrong?" We assured him that there was nothing wrong with the food. We pay the bill and leave in silence. On the way out, I glance at my silhouette in the mirror. A red dress was the wrong attire for this evening.

The drive home is like a return from a funeral. As soon as I open the door, he goes straight to his computer.

"Would you like a drink?"

"I'm fine, thank you," he replies without lifting his head from the screen.

I suffocate in the thick silence, but stay calm and pretend to use my computer as well. Twenty minutes go by without a sound. This is the shutting down Nina warned me about. He finally closes the laptop and heads to the bedroom. I wait a few minutes before joining him. His suitcase is open.

"You're leaving?"

He continues packing. "I changed my flight. I'm leaving tomorrow afternoon."

He still kisses me goodnight but moves to the opposite side of the bed to sleep while I question my reasoning. Moving to Argentina means tackling another challenge: sharing him with the most important person in his life. It's too soon to start a new battle. But losing him is not an option. I lie still on my back and stare at the ceiling shadows cast by the moonlight and forming abstract art of threatening ghosts. Putting my hand on his provokes no reaction. I leave the bed to sit in the kitchen as I used to do when I was little. Whenever I was worried and could not sleep, I'd sit at the kitchen table, joined by Fred—my first therapist. He'd curl up at my feet. The softness of his fur and the warmth of his love soothed any of my rough edges. Sometimes, I sat on the floor to be closer to him. My mother would find us asleep in the morning and scold me for teaching Fred bad habits. "He's a dog!" she'd yell.

I turn off the lights and let the machinery in my brain churn as I await the sunrise. It's 6:30 a.m. when the first rays penetrate the curtains and cast shadows on the kitchen wall.

I dress and run to the bagel bakery.

When I return, I set the table and pour myself a cup of tea. He smiles when he enters the kitchen.

"You've gone to a lot of trouble," he says as he walks by me.

I was hoping he'd come up behind me and hug me as he usually does. He goes straight to the coffee machine, brews himself a cup, and sits down. He eats only half a bagel.

"I need to get an antigen test. There is a lab nearby that opens at 9:00. We need to leave now to avoid waiting in line. After the test, you can drop me off at the airport."

"Daniel, why are you shutting down?"

"You've made a choice that doesn't include me. There is nothing more to discuss."

"So, that's it? You're just gonna walk out?"

"Annie, I don't want to see you for entertainment. I want us to share a life. When you're ready, you know where to find me."

"So, this is a trial breakup?" I try to inject some humor to cut through the heaviness. He sips his coffee and stares at Tony, who's enjoying his breakfast.

"I didn't say no. I just need more time before I shift gears and move to a new country."

"We've been through a lot these past months. If our love wasn't strong enough, it would've ended by now. What more do you need?"

I move closer to hug him. He puts his arms around me but doesn't touch my hair, which he always brushed with his fingers, nor does he run his hand along my back. Uncomfortable, I withdraw.

The closeness we built over the last three days is now shattered; I drive him to the lab and wait in the car.

The drive to the airport is robotic. I follow the highway intuitively. Cars zip by me. He texts his daughter and occasionally smiles at her replies. This is what's waiting for me in Argentina. I sink in my seat and become as shut down as he is.

At the airport, he removes his suitcase from the trunk and hugs me with wooden arms.

"Will you text, so I know you got home safely?"

He bows his head and cracked a smile. "Aerolíneas Argentinas. If it crashes, you'll know I'm in it."

"I can't believe you'd say that to me."

"Take some time to think about what you want. We'll talk soon." He hugs me briskly as if I were a porcupine and flees.

The strength and certitude I so admire about him are now a weapon aimed at me. I drive home with crippling fear stalking me.

Ron is waiting behind the azaleas. "We got a boyfriend, huh?" he says as I exit the car.

"Hi, Ron."

"Where's he from?"

"Argentina."

"I'm happy for you. You're the type of woman… You need a man to treat you special." He wraps his lips around the beer portal.

Λ Λ Λ

Unlike most girls, I never fantasized about a wedding when I was a child. Instead, I dreamed of winning the Nobel Prize. I've been secretly nurturing this dream for years. Starting over in a new country may push this dream even further into the future—if it's even possible at all. Do I have to choose between love and a career? A career is a carefully planned choice. Love is an unexpected turn in the road, like trying for a baby and ending up with twins.

It's been two weeks since he left. No text, no calls. The relationship is slowly shriveling, but I still can't decide. I compose text after text and delete them. I tell myself he's using the power of silence as a strategy to create insecurity, so I'll submit to his will. But I know that's not the case. He's never played any such immature games. He'll come back, I reassure myself. But what if he doesn't? I go back and forth; I negotiate with myself; I make a list of reasons I should contact him, followed by another for why I shouldn't.

I can't give him what he wants just to hold on to him, but my world feels smaller without him. How did I get so weak and let someone occupy so much space in my life? This is the type of woman I counsel. Then I look at all the good things he brings to my life: love, commitment, security, and passion. My mother would say, "Que demande le peuple, Maire-Antoinette?"

I know exactly who to discuss this with.

"Donna, got a minute?"

"Always."

"Daniel proposed," I announce in a flat tone.

"Why don't I feel like saying congratulations?"

"I turned him down."

"Why would you do that?"

"I think he's controlling."

"You're right. Dump the bastard. I'll send you a couple of losers who'll never return your calls, can't commit to a relationship, and stand you up on dates. You'll have a great time."

"I'm serious. He's always making all the decisions."

"Annie, you have a man who's devoted to you and who knows what he wants. What are you afraid of?"

"If I move to Buenos Aires, I'll be totally dependent on him."

"He may lock you in a basement and ransom you to death."

"Exactly!" We burst into a loud laugh. Donna has a way of drawing joy out of people; laughing with her is cathartic.

"I'll come rescue you, and we'll produce a movie called *Set Me Free, Argentina* and we'll have Julia Roberts play you," she squeals.

"You think this is funny."

"I'm going to tell you something you don't wanna hear. You're so tough, you don't want to need anyone. You're afraid of the hold he has on you. But to love is to be vulnerable, Annie. If you don't open up and take a risk, you'll lose him, and you'll deprive yourself of a happiness most of us only dream of."

"True, it frightens me to be under someone's spell like that. So unlike me. I've always been in control during my relationships."

"Because you've never fallen in love before."

"How about my career? It will definitely suffer if I change countries."

"I think it's the opposite. You'll have a broader perspective. You'll gain a multicultural experience, and there are so many branches of psychology you could study and make a contribution to."

Hours later, Donna's words continue to resonate. Am I unreasonable to safeguard my independence? Can I surrender to this relationship without losing myself? I feed the birds and let Tony steal the seeds.

I try to compose an email. Unable to find the right words to tell him how much I love him, I delete paragraph after paragraph. What if I flew to Buenos Aires to surprise him? What if he's through with me? *Enough!*

With trembling fingers, I dial his number. I pace in the living room as the phone rings in Argentina. To my dismay, it goes to voicemail. He's ignoring my call. I hang up and feel that steel ball again, hanging heavy in my mid-section. I throw the phone on the couch, cover my face with both hands, and pull my head to my knees.

Three hours go by without a callback. I distract myself by doing laundry and paying bills, all while keeping vigil on the phone. Unable to bring the tension down, I redial his number. After a couple of rings, he answers with a drowsy voice.

"Annie?" he mumbles.

"How are you?" I ask, shaking.

"Fine. You?"

"Are you sleeping? It's only five o'clock?"

"It's 1:00 a.m. here. I'm in Dubai."

I tighten my grip on the phone and lift my chest. "What are you doing in Dubai?"

"We got a new project."

"Sorry to wake you." I want to hang up, but he continues to talk.

"I'm awake now. What's going on?"

"I... Well, I've been thinking... Um... I'm happier when I'm with you. So, are you still in the market for a wife?"

"Got any on sale?" We both chuckle, and my entire body relaxes and sinks onto the couch.

"I was actually calling to ask you to pick me up at Ezeiza. About to buy a one-way ticket to Buenos Aires."

"Why don't you come here?"

"Seriously? I've never been to the Middle East."

"Well, Dubai is more of an American city. What d'you say? You're coming?"

"Sure. I'll book a flight right away."

"Humm, maybe I'll propose from the top of Burj Khalifa this time."

"What if *I* want to propose?"

"Even better. There is a Gallery Lafayette in downtown Dubai. I want a big rock."

"So, what's it like to be your wife?"

"It's easy. You just obey my instructions..." He cracks up laughing.

"That's not a good sales pitch. Try again."

"Are you sure this is what you want?"

"I'm sure I don't want a life without you in it."

THE END

BEFORE YOU GO...

If you enjoyed this story, **please** drop a review!

I would appreciate it a LOT.

Reviews are my only way to know how I'm doing.
Your feedback lets me know what I'm doing well,
what I might improve, and the stories you enjoy reading.

This link/QR code will bring you
right to the review page.

The Hill of Seven Colors Review

http://www.amazon.com/review/create-review?&asin=B0D1KRPF8X

Thank you in advance for your time.
This is a tremendous favor I'm asking,
and I hope you can help.

ACKNOWLEDGMENTS

My deepest gratitude goes to the writers of **The Next Big Writer** community. Authors John L. Deboer, Marilyn Johnson, and Barry Campbell have generously donated their time and lent their expertise and wisdom to help me grow as a writer.

I offer my sincerest thanks and appreciations to Charles Brass, a writer of science-fiction and fantasy, who mentored me during the entire writing process and has held my hand through the complex tasks of self-publishing. Without his support and mentorship, this book would have taken a lot longer to arrive in your hands.

Thank you to Wilbert Sweet at **Artstation** for his work on the cover. I appreciate your putting up with my crazy, first-time-published demands. (**www.artstation.com/will**)

I would be remiss if I didn't acknowledge the one who's always by my side, through good and tough times and never complains. She gives me all her love without restraints or conditions and never asks for anything beyond food, water and cuddles. That's my beautiful cat, Fleau.

ABOUT THE AUTHOR

Dominique Hoffman is a clinical nutritionist and a trained pastry chef. All the recipes featured in the treatment center, Años Mejores, of her novel, The Hill of Seven Colors, are her own creation.

When she's not bent over her keyboard lost in thought, straining for that one right word, Dominique also enjoys creating recipes, painting (or, well, learning to), speaking a new language, traveling, and playing with her cat Fleau, who thinks they are biologically related.

Visit her website at:
Zizania Productions (www.zizania.com)

You can email her at:
dominique@zizania.com

She is currently working on her next project.

Made in the USA
Middletown, DE
26 September 2024